YOGA FOR HEALTHY BONES

Yoga for Healthy Bones

A WOMAN'S GUIDE

LINDA SPARROWE

WITH YOGA SEQUENCES BY
PATRICIA WALDEN

ADDITIONAL SEQUENCING BY
Annie Carpenter

FOREWORD BY
Susan E. Brown, Ph.D.

Shambhala Boston & London 2004

Shambhala Publications, Inc.
Horticultural Hall
300 Massachusetts Avenue
Boston, Massachusetts 02115
www.shambhala.com

9 8 7 6 5 4 3 2 1

First Edition

Printed in the United States of America

∞ This edition is printed on acid-free paper that meets the American National
Standards Institute Z39.48 Standard.

Distributed in the United States by Random House, Inc., and in Canada by
Random House of Canada Ltd

Interior design and composition: Greta D. Sibley & Associates

Line drawings by Jennifer Devine.

Library of Congress Cataloging-in-Publication Data
Sparrowe, Linda.
Yoga for healthy bones: a woman's guide/Linda Sparrowe with yoga
sequences by Patricia Walden; additional sequencing by Annie Carpenter;
foreword by Susan E. Brown.
p.   cm.
Includes index.
ISBN 1-59030-117-X (pbk.: alk. paper)
1. Yoga. 2. Osteoporosis in women—Popular works. 3. Bones—Diseases—
Prevention—Popular works. 4. Women—Health and hygiene—Popular works.
I. Walden, Patricia. II. Title.
RA781.7 .S646 2004
613.7'046—dc22
2003025262

Contents

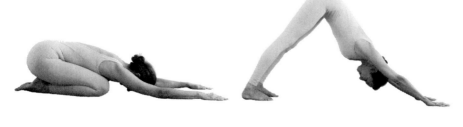

Foreword

EVERY ANIMAL IN THE FOREST EFFORTLESSLY ENJOYS EXCELLENT bone health. Yet, despite considerable effort, millions of humans today experience poor bone health in middle age and beyond. Each year in the United States alone more than 1.5 million fractures occur needlessly. The incidence of osteoporotic fractures in this country continues to rise, despite a federal NIH budget for osteoporosis research that reached $198 million in 2002. Something has gone awry and modern medical science can't seem to find a solution. It appears that all the king's horses and all the king's men cannot put bone health back together again. So what are the king, his horses, his research scientists, and his big health budgets missing?

At the Osteoporosis Education Project we believe that knowledge is the missing element: knowledge not of smaller and smaller bone specifics (which modern science excels at producing), but knowledge about the "big picture"; knowledge about inter-connectedness, about unity, about holism. Our bones are dynamic, constantly changing tissues, connected minute-by-minute to our entire mind-body system. Every morsel we eat, every move we make, and every thought we have affects our bones.

The ancient Indian philosophy of yoga offers a much-needed unified and holistic approach to bone health. This approach has nothing to do with clinical trials or changing scientific opinions. Rather the yoga perspective has everything to do with alignment, balance, harmony, and a life lived in accordance with natural laws. In fact, if you feel tossed about by the seemingly ever-changing reports and recommendations on how to gain and maintain bone health, this book will be a comfort. With admirable simplicity Linda Sparrowe moves us toward unchanging, time-honored ways to renew not only the health of our bones, but also that of our entire body.

In this beautiful and practical book Linda interweaves the wisdom of ancient Eastern traditions with the practical insights of modern Western science to produce a ground-breaking approach to bone health. Gracefully, and with the ease of a journalist, she summarizes current Western medical thought on osteoporosis and bone health. Moving beyond the superficial emphasis on calcium and estrogen, she details a wide range of nutrition and lifestyle factors that can either help or hinder the development and maintenance of strong bones. After establishing this basic groundwork, Linda explores the implications of yoga philosophy and the benefits of yoga postures for bone health.

Linda reminds us of the simple principles of rest and activity. Rest is the basis for activity. Yoga's attention to the breath enlivens our awareness of the principles of giving and receiving. Taking in and letting go are ever-present in our lives as we breathe in and out. Further, these yogic principles of allowing and acceptance free our minds from the fatigue-inducing and bone-damaging clutter of critical thoughts and negative judgments. The Yogis of ancient India proclaimed that life occurs in layers. Indeed, even a cursory inquiry into bone health reveals a multitude of operational layers, nutritional factors, physical forces, electromagnetic forces, hormonal influences, acid-base interactions, and on and on. I have spent two decades investigating the material factors influencing bones. My suspicion, however, has long been that the nonmaterial forces—the nonmaterial layers of life—will prove far more important to bone health than the well-known material forces.

New studies now document the nonmaterial influences on bone. As Linda details, it is now well known that depression and osteoporosis are linked. In fact, any disharmonious emotional or mental state can trigger bone depleting cortisol, adrenaline, and other distress hormones. In a recent Canada-wide bone-health study, Dr. Jerilynn Prior and colleagues asked novel questions about happiness and worry and their relationship to bone health. To the surprise of some, they found that the negative feelings of unhappiness and worry were more highly associated with bone fractures than factors like low calcium intake, lack of exercise, and smoking. These findings provoked me to look up an ancient biblical statement a client shared with me years ago. It's from Proverbs 15:30: "A cheerful look brings joy to the heart, and good news gives health to the bones."

Yoga can help preserve and build bone, I have no doubt. And not just through its physical postures and breathing exercises, but also through the way it quiets the mind as it slows the breath. And not just through the quieting of the mind, but beyond that to the awareness that such stillness promotes an awareness that we are connected to, in union with, the divine life force. Even though surrounded by layers of tumultuous activity, we begin to feel in our center that indeed, all is well in the universe. Allowing ourselves to slip into this profound feeling of well-being will prove, I suspect, to be one of the most important things we can do for our bone health.

Enjoy this book. Take a yoga class. Stretch yourself in many ways and breathe new life into your bones.

Susan E. Brown, Ph.D., C.C.N.
Director of the Osteoporosis Education Project

YOGA FOR HEALTHY BONES

THE SKELETON

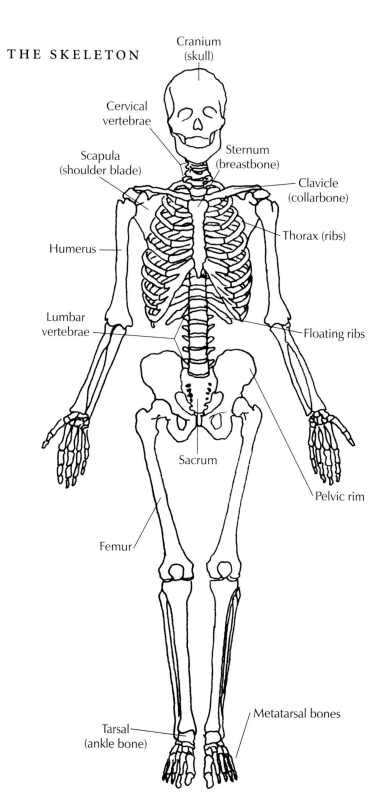

Cranium
(skull)

Cervical
vertebrae

Scapula
(shoulder blade)

Sternum
(breastbone)

Clavicle
(collarbone)

Thorax (ribs)

Humerus

Lumbar
vertebrae

Floating ribs

Sacrum

Pelvic rim

Femur

Tarsal
(ankle bone)

Metatarsal bones

Chapter 1
Getting to Know Your Bones

WHEN WAS THE LAST TIME YOU THOUGHT ABOUT YOUR BONES? When you knocked your shin against that chair leg? When your back "went out" for no apparent reason? More than likely, the only time you focus on your bones is when they hurt. And then you concentrate on relieving the pain and getting back to your daily routine. Your bones deserve better. After all, they're as important to your overall health as the rest of your organs and bodily systems—a fact many of us blithely ignore until we start to ache.

Anyone can experience pain in their joints and bones at any age and anywhere in the body. Ballet dancers complain about problem hips and jammed ankles. Office workers and blue-collar laborers alike try to find relief for lower back pain. Pregnant women often suffer from sciatica, while seniors decry the humpback look and the discomfort of hyperkyphosis (the severe rounding of the thoracic spine known as "dowager's hump"). While injuries, congenital defects, and even immune disorders may contribute to a number of joint and bone complaints, most problems stem from poor posture and weak muscles and are further aggravated by stress, pregnancy, poor nutrition, emotional distress, and overwork.

As we explain in this book, yoga can help you take care of your bones in a number of important ways. First, a daily yoga practice—one that takes your body through its full range of motion—improves your posture and tones your muscles, which reduces abnormal demand on your joints. Second, many poses involve weight-bearing resistance, which increases bone mass. Third, regular practice leads to a more restful sleep and helps reduce your stress level, which can contribute significantly to the health of your bones. Even if your aches and pains stem from a serious degenerative disorder such as osteoarthritis or osteoporosis, a consistent yoga practice, coupled with a sound diet and healthy lifestyle habits, can help stabilize your condition and improve your quality of life.

WHEN SHOULD YOU CARE—AND WHY?

It's never too early—or too late, for that matter—to take care of your bones. Patricia Walden, one of the most widely respected Iyengar yoga teachers in the country, points out that the body you have today is the direct result of what you've done in the past, but the body you will have in the future depends on the habits you cultivate today. And that adage applies to bone health as well. Osteoporosis—bone fractures caused by an abnormal loss of bone mineral density and insufficient peak bone mass (the highest level of bone density you will attain in your lifetime)—may seem like an "old lady's" disease, but the fact is that the stronger your bones are and the better your overall health is during childhood, adolescence, and early adulthood, the less likely you'll be to encounter osteoporotic problems later on. You begin developing your bone mass in infancy—breast-fed babies having a distinct advantage over their bottle-fed counterparts—and you reach peak bone mass by the time you hit thirty. You can influence this bone density level to some extent by eating properly, practicing yoga, and creating a healthy lifestyle. In fact, some doctors say that you can increase bone density by almost 20 percent in your teens and twenties by taking care of yourself, and that should be enough to forestall osteoporosis. But genetics often play a role, too.

Worrying about your bones at eighteen or twenty-five (or forty or fifty) may seem a bit extreme or even hysterical given that osteoporotic fractures may or may not happen until age seventy or older, but osteoporosis is a serious, sometimes fatal problem that affects a large section of the population.

WHAT EXACTLY IS OSTEOPOROSIS?

Osteoporosis literally means "soft or porous bones." There are two types of osteoporosis, which target slightly different populations. Type I, aptly tagged "postmenopausal osteoporosis," affects women who enter their forties and fifties with low peak bone mass and cannot sustain the inevitable 10 to 20 percent drop in bone density that occurs over the five to seven years following the cessation of menstruation. Fractures commonly occur in the wrists and vertebrae of this high-risk group and affect the trabecular bone (the spongy material found inside the cortical bone) more than the hard, outer bone itself.

Type II, or age-associated, osteoporosis is an equal-opportunity affliction, striking both men and women over the age of sixty-five. While type I sufferers experience a rapid decline in bone mass, those with type II osteoporosis lose bone mass gradually over thirty to thirty-five years. This group is likely to face broken hips as well as vertebral fractures that can lead to hyperkyphosis. Type II fractures affect both the trabecular (inner) bone and the cortical (outer) bone.

Both women and men can also suffer from secondary osteoporosis, which means bone fractures are caused by a "foreign" agent or disease, such as hyperthyroidism, hyperparathyroidism, bone tumors, and post-traumatic osteoporosis resulting from injury.

Osteoporotic fractures can occur in one of two ways. The most obvious is from a minor fall in which you break something you normally wouldn't break—like your wrist or your hip. These fractures are obviously painful and require immediate treatment. But there are also "spontaneous fractures," which occur in the vertebrae during normal activities over a period of years and are relatively painless. These "wedge-shaped" fractures compress the spine and decrease height; they also contribute to kyphosis.

Until recently, doctors considered osteoporosis simply an inescapable result of aging, a disease waiting to happen. Now many physicians attribute the disease to a loss of bone mass, which means the body loses more bone cells than it can create. This, they say, causes the bones to become weak and unstable, which increases the risk of fractures. What's the problem with this theory? Every woman, beginning in her thirties, loses more bone than she builds, but not every woman ends up hunched over or suffering from broken bones by age seventy, eighty, or ninety.

Still, the statistics are frightening. According to the U.S. National Osteoporosis Foundation, this silent disease potentially affects 44 million Americans, 80 percent of them women. As the baby boomers finish menopause, an alarming 52 million women will be considered at high risk for osteoporosis, and the number will increase to more than 61 million by the time these women move into their seventies and eighties. Articles in the mainstream press shout more startling statistics:

- One out of every two women in America over the age of fifty will suffer an osteoporotic fracture; 1.5 million such fractures occur every year, including 300,000 broken hips, 700,000 vertebral breaks, and 250,000 wrist fractures.
- Ninety percent of all women over seventy-five have osteoporosis.
- Fifty percent of all women who break a hip because of osteoporosis never walk again, and only 15 percent can walk unaided across the room six months later.

Most doctors caution women that the rapid decrease in estrogen and progesterone after menopause inevitably causes osteoporosis. But, according to Christiane Northrup, M.D., in her landmark book, *Women's Bodies, Women's Wisdom*, blaming osteoporosis on a lack of hormones is too simplistic, especially when statistics indicate that "up to 50 percent of the bone women lose over their lifespan is lost before menopause even begins." She also points out that somewhere between "six and 18 percent of women between 25 and 34 years of age have abnormally low bone density," yet having low (or even abnormally low) bone density doesn't make osteoporotic bone fractures a foregone conclusion. A woman's body doesn't simply self-destruct after menopause because her ovaries inadvertently stop producing the estrogen and progesterone she needs to have healthy bones.

Even though the statistics are frightening, a careful reading of the studies shows that out of the 44 million people who are considered

Patricia Says

To prevent osteoporosis, it's important to incorporate inversions and weight-bearing asanas in your daily practice. Downward-Facing Dog Pose (Adho Mukha Svanasana), Headstand (Sirsasana), and Upward-Facing Bow Pose (Urdhva Dhanurasana) are all beneficial. If you are an advanced practitioner, standing on your hands or doing an elbow balance works well, too. These poses, as well as Upward-Facing Bow Pose, enable you to lift your own weight, which is very important for building bone mass.

"high risk," only 10 million (80 percent of whom are women) actually develop osteoporosis. According to the National Osteoporosis Foundation, 20 percent of all non-Hispanic Caucasian and Asian women over 50, 10 percent of all Hispanic women over 50, and 5 percent of all African-American women over 50 actually have osteoporosis. Although the remaining 34 million women have low bone density indices that place them at risk of osteoporosis, it is important to remember that a low bone mineral density (BMD) reading is an indication of a higher risk factor, not an indication of the disease itself.

Even so, for years doctors prescribed—and women filled prescriptions for—hormone replacement therapy (HRT) with the understanding that an estrogen-progesterone cocktail would provide the only safeguard against this potentially deadly disease. Then in 2001, the Heart and Estrogen/Progestin Replacement Study (HERS), which tracked 2,700 postmenopausal women for four years, determined that HRT proved no more effective than a placebo in protecting women from broken bones. Unfortunately, the study didn't really offer anything promising in place of HRT and left women wondering, "Now what?"

UNAVOIDABLE RISK FACTORS

You can do very little about certain osteoporotic risk factors—they're genetic. If you are very thin with a small frame, for example, you fit the body profile with the highest risk for the disease. Quite simply, your bones aren't as strong and dense as those of a larger boned woman or an average-sized man. Nor can you help it if your mother and her mother endured stress fractures of the vertebrae in their later years, yet that increases your risk as well. So do environmental toxins you may be powerless to escape.

What do all the risk-factor charts point to as the number-one cause of thinning bones? Being a woman. Although Caucasian and Asian women have more of a chance of suffering from osteoporosis than African-American women, all women face greater risk than men. How come? Men, after all, suffer from alcoholism and related conditions more often than women; men also get asthma, take corticosteroidal drugs for pain and inflammation, smoke, eat poorly, and choose the couch over exercise at least as often as we do. What gives? Women, unfortunately, start out with a smaller frame and hence a more delicate bone structure than men; that is, they have less peak bone mass. So when women experience a drastic drop in hormones going through menopause and beyond, they don't have as large a store of bone minerals to rely on. Five years or more after menopause, however, this hormonally induced bone loss levels off. By the time women reach their later years (seventies and eighties), the breaks they experience are probably a result of type II (age-related) or secondary osteoporosis (brought on by other health conditions or diseases). Men are equally susceptible to these types of osteoporosis. In fact, it's almost as common to see an elderly man hunched over with hyperkyphosis (caused by osteoporosis) as it is a woman.

HOW YOGA CAN HELP

No yoga pose will morph a woman into a man, but a consistent yoga practice is what women need to strengthen their bones and keep their adrenals healthy (to produce the level of hormones they need after menopause). The sequence to reverse or prevent bone loss on pages 57–96 will take your body through its full range of motion and offers standing poses as well as balances, backbends, forward bends, inversions, and other asanas to keep you flexible and strong. If you have a small frame and fragile bones, stop smoking, don't drink excessively, and make sure you eat a healthy diet rich in green, leafy vegetables, and whole grains—you need all the help you can get.

RISK FACTORS YOU CAN CONTROL

If low bone density doesn't accurately predict osteoporosis and high levels of calcium don't necessarily prevent it, what does cause your bones to break as you age? Holistic health care providers say that osteoporosis—poor bone quality coupled with low peak bone mass—is a condition created largely by our Western lifestyle. Susan E. Brown, Ph.D., author of *Better Bones, Better Body* and director of the Osteoporosis Education Project in East Syracuse, New York, is a medical anthropologist and a certified nutritionist whose work focuses on the broad cultural perspective of brittle bones. Her research indicates that menopausal women in all cultures lose more bone mass than they build, yet many of these cultures have a very low incidence of osteoporotic fractures. Obviously Western women are doing something wrong. Dr. Brown believes we have "unwittingly developed a diet and lifestyle that wastes calcium and other alkalinizing minerals to the great detriment of our bone health."

Think of your bones as a bank. The more bone mass you have deposited in your account following puberty, the more you have available in your thirties, when bone loss starts to exceed new bone growth. When bone loss accelerates after menopause, your account can sustain these steady withdrawals, because the bone you have left is strong and healthy. However, if you've already "spent" too much bone mass in your youth, this rapid decline can put you at a higher risk for postmenopausal osteoporosis.

Many things contribute to your bone account being overdrawn. Irregular menstrual cycles through your teens and twenties increase your risk for osteoporosis. Young women athletes—track and fielders, ballet dancers, gymnasts—who have intermittent periods often show signs of spinal bone loss even before menopause. So do anorexic girls who no longer have periods because they've stopped ovulating. Diseases of the parathyroid gland affect calcium levels and can place you at risk. Unrelenting stress, a highly acidic diet, mineral deficiencies, and even a lack of exposure to sunlight can contribute to menstrual problems and potentially lead to osteoporosis.

Poor Posture

Poor posture in your early years heightens the risk of developing hyperkyphosis later in life, and this severe rounding of the upper back is a risk factor for osteoporotic fractures. Young women who have tight hamstrings or shoulder muscles, who walk with their heads jutting forward, or who have extreme thoracic scoliosis (curvature of the spine) are prime candidates for hyperkyphosis.

Forward head position, a classic indication of poor self-image and depression, as well as a condition occurring in dedicated couch potatoes and computer operators, can cause kyphosis when left uncorrected. Nursing moms also suffer from the effects of this posture, as do young moms who carry their baby in a backpack. You may think that this condition impacts just your upper back and neck muscles, but jutting your head forward has long-lasting consequences throughout your entire body. Remember that in order to bend, twist, and rotate properly, your spine must be aligned properly. The vertebrae must stack correctly; the cervical, thoracic, and lumbar spines must maintain their curves; and the supporting muscles must relax completely when not in use. When you sit, stand, or walk with your head forward on your neck, lots of things happen. Your upper back and neck muscles immediately tighten in an attempt to hold your head up. Chronically strained upper back and neck muscles can bring on tension headaches or even arthritis in that area. After a while, these same muscles become overstretched and weakened from having to do all that work, which can lead to intervertebral disk problems in your neck and eventual stress fractures. As your head moves out of alignment, your cervical curve decreases, your thoracic curve exaggerates, and your lumbar curve flattens. As your thoracic

Risk Factors for Osteoporosis

- Caucasian or Asian ancestry
- Family history of osteoporosis
- History of excessive or very little exercise
- Amenorrhea (delayed menses)
- Thin, small-boned frame
- History of excessive dieting
- Poor calcium absorption or excessive excretion (determined by blood and urine tests and bone scans)
- Hyperthyroidism
- Smoking
- Clinical depression or high anxiety
- Excessive intake of alcohol, red meat, and caffeine
- Exposure to environmental toxins
- Premature menopause or removal of ovaries before natural menopause
- Use of prescription drugs such as antiepileptic medicine, steroids, and blood thinners

spine rounds, it compromises your ability to twist and rotate your upper back, which puts greater pressure on your lumbar spine to perform those functions.

Forward head position signals the brain that your muscles need help responding to stress, so even your adrenal glands get into the act by producing cortisol, the stress hormone that triggers the fight-or-flight response. Other parts of your body suffer, too. Your shoulder blades move out of alignment, causing rotator cuff problems and inflammation in the surrounding tissues. Your collarbones move forward; your chest collapses inward; and your lungs—lacking adequate space to function—press against your diaphragm, moving it downward against the abdominal wall. Your abdominal muscles weaken, which in turn causes more problems in your lumbar spine.

Forward head position affects you emotionally and mentally as well. You end up focusing on thoughts at the expense of your emotions, literally "leading" with your head and being cut off from bodily sensations. All this because you sit and walk with your head forward!

HOW YOGA CAN HELP

Unless you correct this chronic postural problem, it will only get worse. Yoga can help by addressing the emotional as well as the physical causes of poor posture. Yogis believe that we store much of our emotional pain in the the solar plexus (the area between the heart and the navel); our instinctive desire to protect ourselves also comes from that area of the body. So, if you suffer from poor self-esteem or the "poor me" blues, you have what yogis call "a closed heart," and you try to create a protective barrier around it by rounding your shoulders and allowing your chest to cave inward. Any poses that open up the chest will open your heart and bring you joy. But to successfully counteract the rounded shoulders, compressed diaphragm, and protruding abdomen, you must strengthen your upper back muscles, too.

Standing poses work to correct posture by concentrating on proper alignment and strengthening your core (in and around your navel); they also help take your focus out of your head and move it into your feet, serving to ground your energy. Shoulder and neck openers relax and release the muscles in those areas, allowing the life force (what yogis call *prana*) to move toward the heart region. Backbends open the chest, which increases lung capacity and circulation, and strengthen the back muscles. Inversions rebalance the nervous system. Of course, a daily practice of poses (such as the sequence to reverse or prevent bone loss on pages 57–96) that flex, extend, and rotate your spine is ideal for promoting good posture.

Lack of Exercise

Studies consistently show that exercise increases bone mass in post-menopausal women. The key, according to Kendra Kaye Zuckerman, M.D., director of the osteoporosis program at Allegheny University Hospitals in Philadelphia, is that you must exercise consistently—at least thirty minutes a day, five days a week. Exercise works because it stimulates bone remodeling and improves the absorption of calcium by the bones. Not just any kind of exercise will do, however. Weight-bearing exercise and movements that exert pressure on your bones are what stimulate them to retain calcium. Generally, health care providers recommend walking or running because these exercises stimulate the bones in your feet, legs, pelvis, and spine by combining the effects of gravity and muscle contraction. In contrast, swimming (which can help ease joint pain and increase limited mobility) does nothing to increase bone density.

Yoga is a much better choice for weight-bearing exercise than walking or running because it exerts pressure on all your bones, not just those in your lower body. Handstands and full backbends challenge your fingers, hands, wrists, and shoulders to work together to hold up your body's weight. Headstand (Sirsasana) and Elbowstand (Pincha Mayurasana) stimulate the bones in your elbows and forearms, as well as those in your neck and spine. By taking your spine through its full range of motion, a complete yoga practice improves your posture and keeps the muscles surrounding your bones flexible and strong.

If tests indicate that you've already begun to lose bone mass—and may therefore be susceptible to vertebral stress fractures—you should avoid running because it puts too much stress on your knees, ankles, and lumbar spine. You can continue (or start) practicing yoga, however, because you can modify the poses as needed without diminishing their effectiveness.

One additional caveat about aerobic exercise: Be careful not to overdo it, no matter how young (or old) you are. Excessive exercising and a corresponding drop in body fat can actually increase your chances of osteoporosis, according to the National Osteoporosis Foundation. Young women whose weight has plummeted low enough to cause them to stop ovulating put themselves at risk for the disease later in life.

Anti-Inflammatory Drug Use

Certain drugs increase the risk of osteoporosis. Taking corticosteroids—anti-inflammatory drugs used to manage a variety of diseases such as lupus, asthma, celiac disease, Crohn's disease, ulcerative colitis, and rheumatoid arthritis—can interfere with the bone remodeling process, according to information published by the National Institutes of Health (NIH). The longer you take these drugs (prednisone, cortisone, and others), the more bone density you lose, since they inhibit the absorption of calcium and vitamin D, two critical ingredients for optimal bone health. Corticosteroids also interfere with the production of estrogen and progesterone, which are necessary for bone development. Low levels of these hormones can cause muscle weakness, which increases the risk of falling. Statistics suggest that steroidal drug use is to blame for 20 percent of all osteoporotic fractures.

Asthma

Asthmatics have a high likelihood of osteoporosis for a couple of reasons. First, asthmatics often take corticosteroids to control their asthma, which not only inhibits the absorption of calcium, but also increases its excretion from the kidneys. Second, if you have asthma, you probably don't exercise as much as you should or in a way that would strengthen your bones, because exercise can trigger attacks. Swimming, an exercise doctors often encourage for asthmatics, works wonders for the muscles, but does little to help your bones because it is not weight bearing, like yoga, walking, jogging, volleyball, basketball, or dancing.

HOW YOGA CAN HELP

Asthma actually responds well to yoga practice. In an article in *Yoga Journal*, asthma sufferer and yoga teacher Barbara Benagh quotes Dr.

Learning to Breathe

Tony Sanchez and his wife, Sandy Wong-Sanchez of the U.S. Yoga Association (in San Francisco), created Yogasthma, an asthma management program, in cooperation with Kaiser Permanente and St. Luke's Hospital in San Francisco. The program uses yoga asanas and breathing techniques to help children and their families control their condition. One very important element in their yoga treatment, as in Barbara Benagh's, is relaxation time. Corpse Pose (Savasana) gives the body the deep rest it needs to repair itself and to grow and strengthen. Tony and Sandy suggest that asthmatics focus on the breath and their lungs as they relax completely. As Tony and Sandy like to say, "Smile to yourself; you are in control of your asthma."

Gay Hendricks, author of *Conscious Breathing*, as saying asthma is "more a disturbed breathing pattern than a disease." Because asthmatics tend to overbreathe—that is, inhale too deeply—and not exhale fully enough, Benagh found that she needed to concentrate on shortening her inhalations and lengthening her exhalations and eventually pausing between the two, which helped her slow down her breath. She also feels strongly that you should begin and end the breathing practice with Corpse Pose (Savasana) so you remain deeply relaxed through the whole process.

Yoga postures (asanas) work, too. They can strengthen and relax your chest and back muscles, expand your lungs to increase stamina and respiration, and calm the body. As an asthmatic, you don't have the lung capacity to take advantage of weight-bearing exercises like walking or jogging, but you can do yoga. You'll reap the same benefits from doing a series of slow, deliberate yoga poses in which you breathe steadily and mindfully as you would from a brisk thirty-minute walk.

Yoga also gives you knowledge about your body. Because it connects the breath with the body, you learn more about what triggers an episode and what works to calm you down and lessen the severity of your symptoms.

To create a helpful yoga practice, concentrate on two principles: poses that open up the chest and poses that calm anxiety. In other words, when you are not having symptoms, practice poses such as standing poses and backbends that energize and bring oxygen into your lungs. Also include forward bends, which use the oxygenated breath to calm and restore equilibrium. Do standing poses like Mountain Pose (Tadasana) with various arm positions, Extended Triangle Pose (Utthita Trikonasana) and Half-Moon Pose (Ardha Chandrasana), as well as gentle, supported backbends like Bridge Pose (Setu Bandha Sarvangasana), Reclining Bound Angle Pose (Supta Baddha Konasana), and Camel Pose (Ustrasana), using a chair for support, if necessary. Child's Pose (Adho Mukha Virasana) and Standing Forward Bend (Uttanasana) with your head supported are very relaxing. Always complete your practice with five or ten minutes of Corpse Pose (Savasana).

While yoga won't necessarily allow you to throw away your steroidal inhaler or stop taking those oral corticosteroids, it may lessen the severity of your symptoms enough so you can eventually decrease the dosage and frequency of your medication.

Along with a steady yoga practice, mind what you eat and drink. Increase your intake of fresh fruits and vegetables, drink plenty of water, and stay away from the mucus-producing, sugar-coated foods that may trigger an asthma attack in the first place. Obviously, you don't want to stop any medications without your doctor's advice. But less dependence on this type of medication can translate into fewer osteoporotic fractures later in life.

Digestive Disorders

Those who suffer from irritable bowel conditions (Crohn's disease, ulcerative colitis, irritable bowel syndrome) also fall into the high-risk category for osteoporosis. The Crohn's and Colitis Foundation of America claims 30 to 60 percent of those suffering from these diseases have low bone density, probably because they have difficulty absorbing calcium and vitamin D into the bloodstream from the intestinal tract.

HOW YOGA CAN HELP

A consistent yoga practice can help lessen the painful symptoms of digestive disorders. Ayurvedic physicians trained in the ancient Indian art of holistic healing believe emotional distress contributes to such disorders. They believe emotions, as well as food, can be left in the body "undigested" and contribute to ill health. Repressed anger or resentment, according to Ayurveda, can upset the delicate balance of your gallbladder, bile duct, and small intestines. A restorative practice calms the mind and opens the heart; in doing so, it can help release those pent-up emotions.

Yoga provides the balance between activity and rest that your body needs to function properly. It affords you the opportunity to go inside yourself and notice what your body needs. Certain poses and breathing exercises can also address specific digestive complaints. If your digestive woes accompany perimenopause or postmenopause, pay particular attention to your adrenals, thyroid, and liver, in addition to your belly and intestinal tract. Twists and inversions will help you do this.

If you suffer from too much digestive fire—characterized by bouts of indigestion, acid reflux, or burning sensations after eating—you need postures that will cool your system down. The best poses for this are supported backbends, what Patricia calls "the suptas." These poses lift your diaphragm a bit to take pressure off your stomach. This makes it easier to breathe and gets fresh blood circulating in your abdomen. You don't want to do forward bends if you have a "burning belly" or diarrhea because these poses put too much pressure on your abdomen and create heat. Forward bends do help, however, if you are constipated or bloated. And besides their inherently calming effect on your central nervous system, forward bends exert gentle pressure on your abdomen to help release trapped gas.

Standing poses, if you feel up to doing them, can improve digestion and elimination. You can do these poses with your back against the wall for support, if necessary. Much like supported backbends, these modified poses can cool your digestive system and increase circulation in your abdominal organs.

Adding some twists will help tone and energize your adrenals, liver, and intestines. According to Patricia, even a simple twist can relieve gastritis, and your gallbladder will love the massaging, squeezing effect of twisting poses. This action helps prevent the formation of gallstones and assists in the proper digestion of fat.

Inversions, the quintessential yoga poses, relieve digestive problems in a number of ways. Just by reversing the pull of gravity, they give the abdominal organs—and the nerves supplying them—a break and increase blood flow to the area. Turning upside down is a great way to relieve congestion, improve elimination, and soothe a gassy stomach. It helps balance your endocrine system, particularly your hypothalamus, which controls digestive function, and your thyroid and parathyroids, which govern metabolism; it also calms your central nervous system. A cautionary note, however: Don't confuse your poor digestive system by turning upside down too soon after eating. Always wait at least one and a half to two hours before inverting. And don't practice inversions if you feel nauseous or have a headache.

Ending your practice with Corpse Pose (Savasana) brings you back to your core and enables you to soothe your abdominal organs with the healing power of your breath.

Alcoholism

Alcoholism is yet another risk factor for osteoporosis because it disrupts the mineral balance in the body. A full 98 percent of the calcium you take into your body goes to your bones with your blood and teeth taking up the other 2 percent. The amount of calcium found in your blood depends not only on how much you ingest, but also how much gets absorbed properly and how much gets excreted. Alcoholics seldom get enough nourishment from the food they eat—they often fill up on junk food and alcohol, which makes them mineral deficient. If the body can't get enough calcium and other minerals to function properly, it will "borrow" from the bones, leaving the bones brittle and thin and susceptible to breaks. Some studies suggest that too much alcohol in the bloodstream may actually inhibit the bone-building process.

Chronic drinking can also elevate parathyroid hormone (PTH) levels in the body, which signals the bones to release too much calcium into the bloodstream. Blood calcium levels then rise excessively, which in turn has deleterious effects on the arteries leading to the heart.

Prolonged alcoholism also damages the liver, kidneys, and digestive tract, which makes absorbing and processing food-based minerals more challenging. Too much alcohol can impair balance and the ability to walk, so alcoholics tend to lose their balance and fall more often than most people. In the 2002 Framingham Osteoporosis Study at Tufts University in Boston, researchers concluded that women and men who drink heavily have an increased risk of hip fracture. Also, although vertebral fractures in women under fifty years of age are rare, if you abuse alcohol, the possibility of these types of fractures increases.

Although yogis don't profess to cure alcoholism, many treatment centers now offer twice-weekly or even daily classes as an adjunct therapy to balance the nervous system and reduce cravings and anxiety.

Alcohol abuse and overuse increase the risk of osteoporosis, but an occasional cocktail or a single glass of wine in the evenings may actually slow bone loss in postmenopausal women (but not in those who are pre- or perimenopausal). According to the National Resource Center of the National Institutes of Health, alcohol apparently enhances the conversion of testosterone into estradiol. Estradiol, a form of estrogen, helps maintain bone density. Moderate drinking also increases calcitonin, a thyroid hormone that inhibits bone resorption (the breaking down of bone to capture extra calcium). The good news for excessive drinkers? According to the NIH, once you stop drinking, bone-building activities quickly resume, and some lost bone may be partially restored.

Smoking

As if there weren't enough reasons to quit, studies now show a strong correlation between poor bone health and cigarette smoking. One 1994 Australian study concluded that women who smoked one pack of cigarettes daily throughout adulthood would have a deficit of 5 to 10 percent in bone density by the time they reached menopause, which is enough to increase the risk of fractures. The study began with the premise that cigarette smoking increases the risk of vertebral, forearm, and hip fractures. It looked at sets of female twins—one twin smoked at least five pack-years more than the other (a pack-year is the number of packs of cigarettes one smokes per day, per year). The twins who smoked more heavily had lower bone density at the neck, upper thoracic spine, and lumbar spine. Researchers found a decrease in serum concentrations of PTH and calcium, as well as a greater amount of calcium excreted from the kidneys, an indication that calcium was being leached from the bones.

Although researchers don't know for sure why cigarette smoking causes low bone density, one reason could be that smokers have a more difficult time absorbing nutrients from the foods they eat. Malabsorption of calcium, magnesium, vitamin D, and other vitamins and minerals from foods can cause the body to search for other suppliers, such as the bones. According to the August 1984 issue of the *Journal of the American Medical Association (JAMA)*, cigarette smoking appears to lower the amount of estrogen in the bloodstream and, since estrogen slows the bone-destroying abilities of osteoclasts (see chapter 2), less estrogen means softer bones. John Lee, M.D., a strong proponent of progesterone therapy for menopausal problems, thinks that cigarette smokers don't exhale adequate amounts of carbon dioxide, which may affect bone health. A buildup of carbon dioxide creates excess carbonic acid. In order to neutralize the acid, Dr. Lee says the body must borrow calcium from the bones.

HOW YOGA CAN HELP

Yoga alone can't stop the urge for nicotine, but it can help. One smoking theory postulates that smoking helps lift the spirits of those who battle depression. Standing poses and backbends can do the same thing. If a daily smoking habit calms your anxiety, try forward bends or supported inversions instead. Many women, after doing yoga consistently for several months, reported that they no longer wanted to defile their body by infusing it with nicotine; others felt the practice of asanas and pranayama (breathing exercises) worked better than the over-the-counter quit-smoking remedies they'd tried. "Practicing yoga, even a few minutes of concentrated breathing, stopped me from reaching for that next cigarette," said Caroline, a magazine editor with a ten-year, pack-a-day habit.

Depression

The latest research suggests that depression in premenopausal women is a significant risk factor for osteoporosis. This rather discouraging piece of news further implicates depression as a serious health problem with long-term effects. The U.S. Center for Mental Health Services suggests that at least 5 percent of American adults suffer from depression annually. Other researchers believe it's more like 20 percent. In *Women's Bodies, Women's Wisdom*, Christiane Northrup estimates that at least a quarter of all women in the United States battle serious depression sometime in their lives.

Most women think of depression as incapacitating: The world presses down on them; there's a weight on their chest; their breathing feels shallow; they've lost the ability or desire to do anything. This is one type of depression (chronic); it grips your entire being and leaves you feeling as empty as a deflated balloon. But thousands of women suffer from another, equally insidious type of depression that is masked by high levels of anxiety and is thus called anxiety-driven depression. Their high-stress lifestyle keeps them from experiencing the feelings beneath their tension and fear; it keeps them from recognizing what's really going on inside. They feel anxious all the time and find themselves easily agitated, quick to anger, and very impatient.

If you already have a yoga or meditation practice, you know that all these emotions—sadness, despair, anxiety—affect more than your mental state. They manifest in the body as menstrual irregularities, digestive disorders, or even chest pains. Going deeper still, chronic depression or anxiety takes its toll on your nervous system, too.

So, how does all this sadness and anxiety lead to brittle bones? If your depression relates to hormonal fluctuation (either after pregnancy or during perimenopause), a drop in estrogen levels could be the culprit.

Too little estrogen has a negative effect on bone density, so as a side effect, hormonally charged depression could cause the body to build bone inefficiently. Both the thyroid and the parathyroid glands help regulate the amount of calcium in the bloodstream, so hypothyroidism—a condition that brings on both depression and fatigue—also upsets the way the body makes bone.

Elevated levels of the stress hormone cortisol appear to play a major role in depression-related osteoporosis (see chapter 3). In a 1996 study funded by the National Institute of Mental Health (NIMH), researchers found—among other indicators—higher than normal urinary cortisol levels in women with past or current depression. High levels of cortisol, a hormone produced by the adrenal glands, may depress the body's ability to build bone. Although a new NIMH study is in the works to better understand the correlation between depression and bone loss, researchers now believe that cortisol plays a role, that depression impairs calcium absorption, and that other hormone deficiencies may contribute to low bone density.

Depression won't cause brittle bones unless you have other risk factors as well—small frame, low peak bone mass, anovulatory periods—or you smoke or drink excessively. But the NIMH study's findings that the decrease in bone density was significant in twenty-four otherwise healthy premenopausal women (more than 13 percent at the neck and almost 11 percent at the hip) suggest that depression-related bone loss could increase your lifetime risk of fracture by as much as 50 percent.

HOW YOGA CAN HELP

Even novice yoga practitioners say that it's impossible to separate the physiological benefits of yoga from the emotional and spiritual ones. After all, as Patricia says, thoughts affect feelings, which in turn affect physiology. In yoga, the reverse is also true. For example, Inverted Staff Pose (Viparita Dandasana) is a back-bending chest opener. The mere act of lifting your chest can elevate your emotions and lead your mind to a clearer state. It creates space for your breath to move more freely, and freer breath brings lighter feelings. Backbends further release any blockage in and around your heart that could be contributing to your rounded shoulders and sunken chest.

Seated forward bends, on the other hand, can quiet a nervous system that goes into overdrive when you become anxious or fearful. These poses provide an invaluable antidote to cortisol overload. Inversions allow oxygenated blood to circulate more freely, which soothes and then energizes the glands in and around your head and throat. Standing poses can also elevate your mood, making you feel stronger and more capable (literally, "standing on your own two feet").

Corpse Pose (Savasana) and other restorative poses provide conscious rest for your sympathetic nervous system—and your whole body—so healing can take place. They induce a state of complete relaxation, so your brain can restore itself and rebalance its neurotransmitters. They also give you an opportunity to look deeper inside and discover where the tensions lie or where the pain resides, and they send the gift of breath to help push some of the tension and pain out.

Yoga reminds you that nothing is permanent, that you are not your feelings. By staying present in a pose, especially one that challenges you at first, you learn that you can be uncomfortable, even unhappy, and still be all right. As your proficiency increases, you come to see that what was impossible last week is doable today.

Working with your breath in the physical poses and during breathing practice (pranayama) can be a wonderful aid. Patricia says that deep, healing inhalations lift your spirits and long, slow exhalations soothe your nerves. Don't be surprised if feelings of sadness, anger, or even fear well up inside you during your practice. Acknowledge them and then let them go. They've been waiting to get out for a long time.

Do the practice found on pages 34–52 as often as your schedule allows. But try to do at least something every day—ten minutes of Corpse Pose (Savasana), for example—in order to heal your spirit and counteract the effects your moods have on your body.

Chapter 2
The Physiology of Bone

BEFORE YOU CAN UNDERSTAND HOW TO PREVENT OR POSSIBLY EVEN reverse bone loss, it helps to know a bit about the bone-making process and to start thinking about your bones as living, ever-changing tissue. Your bones are strong yet flexible. The outer cortex, or sheath of the bone, is hard; inside is a spongy tissue resembling a honeycomb. Called the trabecular bone, this matrix is made up of fibers filled with crystalline minerals—primarily calcium and phosphorus—and collagen protein. The minerals make the bone hard; the collagen gives bone its strength and flexibility. The spaces within the honeycomb contain blood vessels and the soft bone marrow that manufactures your blood cells.

Your body breaks down and rebuilds trabecular bone constantly through an intricate dance between osteoclasts (bone breakers) and osteoblasts (bone makers) choreographed by the female hormones estrogen and progesterone, and accompanied by testosterone, parathyroid hormone, adrenals, and the thyroid hormone calcitonin.

Osteoclasts remove minerals and protein from the bones and release them into the bloodstream in a process called bone resorption. Osteoblasts replace them. First the osteoblasts secrete collagen to remake the matrix that the osteoclasts have destroyed. Then they seek out new sources of vitamins A, C, D, and K, and minerals like calcium, magnesium, phosphorus, manganese, zinc, boron, copper, and silicon to add into the protein matrix to form new bone. The healthier the matrix, the stronger and more resilient the bones.

Patricia Says

- Maintain good posture, with your head over your shoulders and your shoulders in line with your hips, to prevent pressure on your spine. Practice sitting, standing, and walking with the same posture you use in Mountain Pose (Tadasana).
- Put your body through its full range of motion—from standing to sitting, right side up and upside down, back and forth, and twisting side to side—to increase and maintain mobility and flexibility.
- Incorporate restorative poses that allow your body and your muscles to relax completely.

Estrogen, which predominates during the first half of your menstrual cycle, stimulates your bones to retain calcium. Estrogen also exerts some control over how much bone you lose by slowing the action of the bone-wrecking osteoclasts. Progesterone, on the other hand, stimulates bone-building osteoblasts. Because progesterone is manufactured in your ovaries during the second phase of your cycle, you need to ovulate in order to build new bone efficiently. If you don't ovulate regularly, you'll lose bone mass faster than you build it, which shouldn't happen until you reach your early thirties.

All this bone making and breaking has an important goal: to ensure that your body has adequate levels of calcium to function properly. Your body needs calcium to regulate its heartbeat and the flow of its nerve impulses and for critical blood-clotting functions. The strength of your muscles and bones, and even your teeth and gums, depends on calcium, which you also need to contract your muscles.

Hormones from your parathyroid and thyroid glands work to regulate your metabolism and ensure that your body gets the calcium and vitamin D it needs. The parathyroid gland is specifically designated as the body's calcium regulator. If you ingest enough calcium, the parathyroid instructs your bones to store the excess and use it to make new bone; if you lack calcium, the parathyroid gland instructs your kidneys to keep their reserves on hold; it also signals the osteoclasts to break down more bone and release the needed calcium into your bloodstream. If, over time, you fail to take in enough calcium, your bones will run a calcium deficit, which will cause them to become softer and more porous. The adrenal glands manufacture steroid hormones (the ones that respond to physical stress), which help your bones give up calcium in an emergency (bone resorption). Testosterone and other androgens (which your adrenals manufacture after menopause) promote bone growth to balance the bone-resorbing action of the steroid hormones.

From early infancy through puberty, your body builds more bone than it breaks down. In your twenties, the action of osteoclasts and osteoblasts evens out and you achieve your peak bone mass. After thirty, the osteoclasts break down bone much faster than their counterparts build it, and you begin to loss bone mass. If you have taken care of yourself through diet, exercise, and good lifestyle habits, you'll have a storehouse of strong, healthy bones (your peak bone mass will have been high) and you can afford to withdraw the calcium your body needs, as long as these withdrawals are moderate and infrequent. However, if you enter your thirties with low bone mass, or if your lifestyle dictates that your bones must give up inordinate amounts of calcium and other minerals, your bones can become brittle and your risk for osteoporosis can skyrocket. Does that mean your fate is sealed if you're over thirty? Not necessarily. Even if you haven't paid much attention to your bones until now, don't despair. It's never too late to start.

DIET AND THE CALCIUM CONUNDRUM

If all we needed to prevent osteoporosis were plenty of calcium and additional estrogen, American women—who drink more milk and take more hormone supplements than any other women in the world— would have the lowest rate of osteoporosis. They don't; they have among the highest. Counterintuitively, women in countries that have the lowest rate of osteoporosis consume the least amount of calcium. Some research even suggests that ingesting too much calcium is as detrimental to the health of your bones and heart as ingesting too little. That doesn't seem possible until you understand that your body has to be able to use the calcium you take in through food or vitamin supplements. If you don't have enough vitamin D, magnesium, potassium, iron, and other minerals in your diet, all of which are critical cofactors for moving calcium into the bone, your body can't absorb calcium efficiently. And if it can't absorb something, your body can't use it. Unfortunately, that's not all. Unabsorbed calcium doesn't just flush harmlessly through the body and get excreted in the urine. Some of it stays in the body where it can show up in your joints (arthritis and fibromyalgia), in your arteries (heart disease), and in your kidneys (kidney stones).

Another compelling theory says that American women need to take more calcium and its cofactor minerals because of our diet and lifestyle choices. Susan E. Brown, Ph.D., says we need more because "we have a lot of calcium-wasting things in our diets—high levels of protein and phosphoric acid, for example." Here are some bone-friendly suggestions that should help you get the most from your diet.

Eat Less Animal-Derived Protein

Research shows that vegetarian women lose far less bone mass than their meat-eating sisters. In fact, one study conducted in southwestern Michigan reported that women who were vegetarians for twenty years lost only 18 percent of their peak bone mass over the course of the study, while their carnivorous counterparts suffered 35 percent loss. One reason for that, according to Dean Ornish, M.D., director of the Preventive Medicine Research Institute in Sausalito, California, is that a diet high in animal protein can cause your body to excrete too much calcium through urine. That means your body actually gets rid of the calcium before you can benefit from it. Vegetarians, on the other hand, excrete far less calcium and therefore profit from its bone-strengthening properties.

Eat an Alkaline Diet

Too much animal protein also produces an excess of phosphorus, which the body converts to phosphoric acid. According to Susan Brown, your body can buffer about 50 to 60 grams of protein every day; if you eat more than that (and most Westerners eat as much as 100 grams), the excess amino acids (by-products of protein) stay in the bloodstream and render your blood too acidic. If you eat lots of fruits and vegetables high in alkaloids (that is, chock full of calcium, magnesium, iron, and potassium), your body can neutralize that excess acid and return to the slightly alkaline state that is so critical to good health. On the other hand, if you drink lots of soda, which is high in phosphoric acid, and eat processed cheese, fried foods, and snack foods laden with aspartame (artificial sweetener), your body will need to find more acid neutralizers. So it first searches for sodium and potassium buffers in the body. Once it depletes those reserves, according to Dr. Brown, the body pulls calcium and magnesium and other minerals from the bones, which weakens them.

You still need adequate amounts of protein for healthy bones, since the trabecular bone matrix that holds the minerals comes from protein. But if you eat animal protein, Dr. Brown advises balancing it with increased potassium, which you will find in bananas, cantaloupe, fresh orange juice, almonds, Swiss chard, and artichokes.

If you eat a healthy, more alkaline diet, your body won't have to turn to the acid-neutralizing minerals in your bones as often. Some of the most alkaline foods, according to Dr. Brown, include pumpkin seeds, lentils, yams, limes, nectarines, persimmons, raspberries, tangerines, pineapples, dark leafy vegetables, and spices like cinnamon.

Be Calcium Smart

Adequate amounts of calcium—the recommended daily amount (RDA) is 1,000 mg/day before and during menopause and 1,500 mg/day after menopause—are critical to healthy bones and a healthy heart. To avoid potential problems from too much calcium, remember that the RDA equals the total amount you take in to your body from food sources as well as supplements, not from supplements alone.

Despite the RDA, the jury's still out on how much calcium is enough. One study, published in a 1998 article in *Internal Medicine News*, found that taking 1,200 to 1,500 mg/day of calcium and 700 to 800 IU/day of vitamin D supplements reduced fractures in postmenopausal women by 50 percent. On the other hand, Nan Kathryn Fuchs, Ph.D., in her very useful booklet *User's Guide to Calcium & Magnesium*, cites one Mayo Clinic study in particular, which suggests that it makes no difference whether you take 1,400 mg/day of calcium or only 500 mg. The rate of bone loss is the same.

According to David Levinson, M.D., of the Cornell University Medical Center, your body can't handle much more than 500 mg of calcium at a time; so if you do take a 1,000-mg supplement, take 500 mg in the morning and 500 mg at night.

There are many good food-based sources of calcium besides milk. Dr. Fuchs says all dairy products "are high in calcium, but they don't have enough magnesium in them to help move it into your bones." You can get adequate calcium, along with its cofactors (vitamins A, B_6, C, D, and E and magnesium and other trace minerals) from a variety of sources—dark green leafy vegetables, carrots, almonds, tofu, miso and other soy products, seaweed, and salmon. Drink calcium-enriched orange juice—one glass delivers as much calcium as a glass of milk. Good calcium-rich herbs include nettles, horsetail, sage, oatstraw, borage, raspberry leaf, and alfalfa.

If you take calcium supplements, be sure to follow the directions on the label for maximum absorption. Some supplemental calcium, like calcium carbonate, gets absorbed better with food; other types, like calcium citrate, work better on an empty stomach. To use the calcium you do take in, your body needs adequate amounts of all those other vitamins and minerals, but it also needs enough hydrochloric (or stomach) acid—which postmenopausal women often lack. If you have that problem, you can purchase betaine hydrochloric acid at your local health food store. Or, you may find taking calcium with acidic foods or with a glass of orange juice helps your body absorb it more readily. Current studies show that calcium citrate malate may be the most easily absorbed. (Note: Don't try to get your calcium from antacids that contain aluminum, which causes the calcium to be excreted.)

Beware of Calcium Robbers

Too much salt can leach calcium from your bones, just as too much protein can. Watch out for hidden salt in processed foods and canned goods. Phosphates in carbonated soft drinks can also steal from your body's calcium supply, as can caffeine, alcohol, and nicotine. Some researchers warn that consuming more than three cups of caffeinated coffee a day can increase your risk factor for bone loss by 80 percent. Cigarette smoking and even moderate alcohol consumption double your risk. Sugar consumption causes big problems, too. The 2002 Framingham Osteoporosis Study at Tufts University in Boston demonstrated that a diet high in sugar content was the single most reliable predictor of low bone mineral density in older men and women. Sugar upsets the acid-alkaline balance in the body, causing your body to leach calcium from your bones. Consider giving up your sugar habit!

Sunbathe

Everyone knows the dangers of getting too much sun. However, the body needs sunlight to produce vitamin D. Twenty-five to thirty minutes four or five times a week should give you all the vitamin D your body needs to absorb and use calcium effectively. If you are ultrasensitive to direct sun, add vitamin D to your daily supplements instead. Recent studies point to the importance of adequate vitamin D in overall bone health and to the health of your reproductive glands and your entire immune system. Some promising studies suggest that vitamin D can actually reduce the risk of fractures by a third (in comparison, certain medications, such as estrogen or progesterone therapy, claim to reduce fractures by 50 percent).

Additional Supplements

Besides taking enough calcium, magnesium, and vitamin D, increasing your vitamin K intake may help your bones stay strong, according to

researchers at Tufts University. If you're not on blood-thinning medication (such as coumadin), ask your doctor whether increasing your daily
intake of vitamin K makes sense. It's actually easy (and preferable) to get
all you need from the food you eat. Just one-half cup of collard greens,
for example, provides more than 400 mcg of vitamin K; the same
amount of spinach yields 360 mcg; and broccoli packs 113 mcg into that
little half cup. Essential fatty acids, vitamins B_6 and C, and folic acid also
contribute to good, healthy bone structure.

Magnesium plays a critical role in optimal calcium absorption and
good bone health. It helps move calcium into the protein matrix of the
bone and balances the effect calcium has on the muscles. Whereas calcium
contracts muscle, magnesium relaxes it. The right balance of calcium and
magnesium then helps the heart and other muscles, as well as the digestive system, function properly.

Women need approximately 2 mg of copper, 3 mg of manganese, and
12 mg of zinc every day. Nuts, berries, tofu, and tomatoes provide
enough manganese and copper; seafood and peas are good sources of
zinc. Other trace minerals also enhance calcium's ability to increase
bone density, and boron seems to help as well. While scientists aren't ex-
actly sure how beneficial it is, studies now show that boron aids in the
metabolism of calcium, phosphorus, and vitamin D. Since high urinary
concentrations of calcium and phosphorus indicate absorption problems, make sure you get at least 3 mg of boron a day.

Chapter 3
The Cortisol Connection

WE OFTEN THINK OF STRESS AS JUST ANOTHER BY-PRODUCT OF OUR fast-paced culture, something we encounter at work or when we're over-scheduled at home. But more and more studies are finding that stress plays an important and negative role in numerous diseases, including osteoporosis. The culprit seems to be cortisol, the stress hormone implicated in anxiety and chronic depression. Cortisol itself provides a necessary service in the body as one of the instigators of the fight-or-flight response—the mechanism the body uses to escape danger. Problems occur when your body stays stuck in that response.

If you've ever stepped off the curb and barely missed being hit by a car, you know what this response feels like. Your adrenaline soars, your blood pressure rises, your heart pounds wildly, you sweat like crazy, your mind goes on hyperalert, and your breath becomes shallow and quick. To bring as much power as possible to your sympathetic nervous system (which controls this response) so you can react quickly and efficiently, your body diverts energy from your digestive, reproductive, and immune systems, slowing them down to a bare maintenance level. It does this by activating what is called the hypothalamic-pituitary-adrenal (HPA) axis, or "stress circuit." Here's how it works. When you step off that curb and first see the speeding car, your brain immediately signals your nervous system's HPA axis to release stress hormones into your bloodstream so you can jump out of the way. The hypothalamus releases corticotropin-releasing hormone (CRH), which in turn triggers the pituitary gland to pour adrenocorticotropic hormone (ACTH) into the bloodstream. By doing this, the pituitary gland sends a warning to the adrenals, which then respond by releasing an army of hormonal compounds—epinephrine (adrenaline), norepinephrine, and cortisol. Epinephrine and norepinephrine cause your blood pressure to rise; epinephrine also increases your heart rate, diverts blood into your large muscle groups (in your arms and legs), and speeds up your reaction time. Cortisol, formally called glucocorticoid, releases sugar (fuel) into your bloodstream so you can think and move faster and suppresses insulin production. With your heart, brain, and large muscle groups on high alert, the HPA axis continues to communicate with the rest of your body, instructing your digestive, reproductive, and immune systems to slow down and wait out the danger.

Once you realize you're safe, cortisol signals the hypothalamus that all is well and instructs it to stop producing CRH. You begin to calm down, and your nervous system goes back to normal. In other words, the stress circuit switches off. But what happens if you don't calm down, if you continue to live your life in hyperstress mode? The HPA axis remains in fight-or-flight mode, never giving your nervous system a chance to return to a balanced state. As a result, your adrenal glands become exhausted from constantly pumping stress hormones into your body; your digestive and immune systems remain sluggish; and the neurotransmitters that signal a feeling of well-being are seriously lacking. Eventually, immune surveillance can shut down, creating an opening for opportunistic viruses and bacteria to enter your body and do serious damage.

According to George Chrousos, M.D., chief of pediatric and reproductive endocrinology at the National Institute of Child Health and Human Development, the stress response works differently in everyone. Some people trigger the fight-or-flight response at the slightest provocation; others may not respond quickly or urgently enough. Environmental toxins can inhibit HPA responses; alternatively, Dr. Chrousos says that too much stress in childhood can actually create a stronger HPA feedback loop so that, as you age, you may find yourself overreacting to the simplest problem. Some research even suggests that continual stress can impair your body's ability to switch off the stress response during times of relative calm.

As a woman, you may be more susceptible to stress and have higher cortisol levels in your bloodstream than men. Cortisol and other corticosteroid hormones, if they hang around at elevated levels too long, can inhibit the production of estrogen and progesterone, the essential hormones not only for reproduction, but for bone health as well.

HOW YOGA CAN HELP

Yoga can mitigate stress and counter the effects of these stressor hormones on the central nervous system through a combination of active asanas (poses), pranayama (conscious breathing), and deep relaxation. A few small studies confirm what most yoga practitioners already know: yoga works. Eric Hoffman, Ph.D., conducted a Scandinavian study in which he showed that alpha waves (which measure relaxation) and theta waves (which measure dreams, unconscious memory, emotions, and deep states of relaxation) increased by 40 percent after a two-hour yoga class. The National Institute of Mental Health and Neurosciences in India performed six studies on the benefits of Sudarsham Kriya yoga, a series of deep-breathing techniques, and found it to be at least as effective as conventional treatments in treating stress-related disorders. The study also noted a beneficial drop in stress-hormone levels. Participants in a Philadelphia study experienced a significant drop in cortisol levels after only one yoga class.

None of these studies comes as any surprise to seasoned yoga practitioners. B. K. S. Iyengar, a master of yoga's therapeutic applications, believes that certain yoga poses quiet your sympathetic nervous system (the fight-or-flight instigator), replenish your adrenals when they have been working overtime, and promote a general feeling of well-being. Patricia notes that forward bends using a bolster or chair (so your back muscles do less work) produce a feeling of literally being supported, of being safe from outside stressors.

Do the following practice as often as your schedule allows. But try to do at least something every day—ten minutes of Corpse Pose (Savasana), for example—in order to heal your spirit and counteract the effects of cortisol on your body.

A SEQUENCE TO MITIGATE STRESS AND
RELIEVE DEPRESSION

1. Cross Bolsters Pose or Reclining Easy Seated Pose (Supta Sukhasana)
2. Downward-Facing Dog Pose (Adho Mukha Svanasana)
3. Half-Moon Pose (Ardha Chandrasana)
4. Headstand (Sirsasana)† or Wide-Angle Standing Forward Bend (Prasarita Padottanasana)
5. Camel Pose (Ustrasana)
6. Downward-Facing Dog Pose (Adho Mukha Svanasana) or Child's Pose (Adho Mukha Virasana)
7. Shoulderstand (Sarvangasana)† or Bridge Pose (Setu Bandha Sarvangasana)
8. Half-Plough Pose (Ardha Halasana)†
9. Bridge Pose (Setu Bandha Sarvangasana)
10. Corpse Pose (Savasana)

†CAUTION You may want to skip or modify these poses due to health limitations or ability. Please read the explanatory footnote beneath the descriptions before giving them a try.

1. CROSS BOLSTERS POSE Place a bolster on your mat and lay another one across the center of the first to form a cross. Sit on the middle of the top bolster. Using your hands on the floor to guide you, carefully lie back so your spine is supported on the bolster and the back of your head touches the floor. (If that is too much of a stretch or puts strain on your neck, place a folded blanket underneath your head.) Place your arms on either side of your head, palms up, elbows bent, and relax completely. (If you feel any strain or tension in your lower back, raise your feet on a block.) Relax in this pose for several minutes, softening your abdominals and breathing deeply. To come out of the pose, bend your knees and roll to one side. Use your hands to help yourself up to a seated position. If this pose creates too much of a backbend for you and causes any discomfort, practice Reclining Seated Pose (Supta Sukhasana) instead.

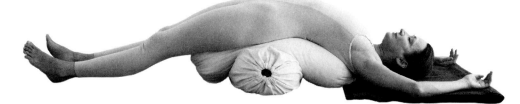

ALTERNATIVE: RECLINING EASY SEATED POSE (Supta Sukhasana) Place a bolster vertically on the floor behind you and sit just in front of it with your knees bent and your sacrum touching the bolster's edge. You may put a folded blanket on the bolster to support your head. Cross your legs comfortably at your shins and extend up through your spine. Using your hands to support you, lie back on the bolster. Rest your arms out to the sides, bring your shoulder blades into your back ribs, and lift your chest. This should be a restful pose and you should feel no discomfort anywhere. (If you feel any strain in your back, add more height to your support.) To come out, uncross your legs, place your feet flat on the floor, and roll slowly to one side. Use your hands to push yourself up to a sitting position.

EFFECTS Both of these supported backbends open your chest, improve respiration and circulation, help balance adrenal and thyroid function, and help alleviate depression and fatigue.

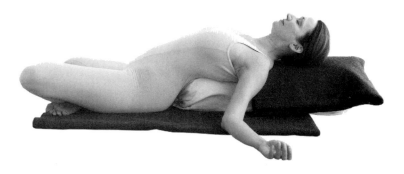

2. DOWNWARD-FACING DOG POSE (Adho Mukha Svanasana) Lie facedown on your sticky mat. Place your palms on the floor by each side of your chest with your fingers well spread and pointing straight ahead. Come up on your hands and knees. That's your position. Now place a bolster or a folded blanket or two vertically so your support is in line with your sternum. Your support should be high enough to support your head, but low enough to lengthen your neck. Return to your hands-and-knees position and turn your toes under.

Exhale, press your hands firmly into the mat and extend up through your inner arms. As you exhale, raise your buttocks high into the air and move your thighs up and back. Keep stretching through your legs and bring your heels toward the floor. Keep your legs firm and your elbows straight as you lift your buttocks upward and release your head onto your support. The action of the arms and legs serves to elongate your spine and release your head. Hold this pose for 30 seconds to 1 minute, breathing deeply. Let your head rest completely and release the base of your neck. To come out, return to your hands and knees and sit back on your heels.

EFFECTS This is a wonderful pose to combat depression because it helps increase circulation to your chest, improve respiration, and calm your brain.

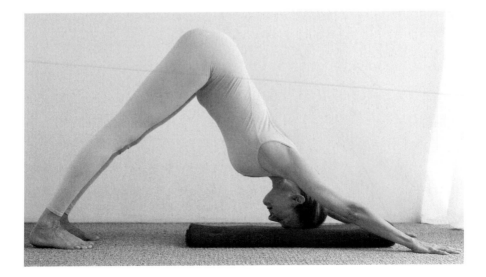

3. HALF-MOON POSE (Ardha Chandrasana) With your back toward a wall, step your feet about 3½ feet apart. Turn your left foot out 90 degrees and your right foot slightly inward. Line up the heel of your left foot with the arch of your right. Place a block at the outside edge of your left foot. Stretch your arms out and lift your abdomen and chest. Exhale, extend your trunk to the left, and bring your left hand down to the block. Bend your left knee and move the block about a foot in front of your left leg. Raise your right foot off the floor and come up onto your toes. Exhale, straighten your left leg, raise your right leg parallel to the floor, and press your left heel down. Your right leg, hips, shoulders, and head now rest against the wall. Stretch your right arm up in line with your shoulders and open your chest and pelvis. Draw your shoulder blades into your back and look up or straight ahead. Hold for 15 seconds. To come down, bend your left leg, reach your right leg back, and put your foot on the floor, moving the block with you. Inhale, stand up, and repeat on the other side.

EFFECTS This pose helps you open your chest and energize your whole body, without worrying about balance.

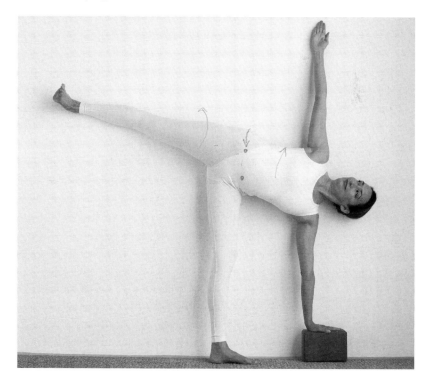

4. HEADSTAND† **(Sirsasana)** Place a folded blanket against the wall. Kneel in front of it with your feet and knees together. Interlace your fingers firmly, thumbs touching and your hands cupped. Position your hands no more than 3 inches from the wall, your elbows shoulder-width apart. Your wrists, forearms, and elbows form the foundation for this pose.

Lengthen your neck and place the crown of your head on the blanket. The back of your head should be in contact with your hands. Press your forearms into the floor and lift your shoulders away from the floor. Maintain this action throughout the pose. Straighten your legs, raise your hips toward the ceiling, and walk your feet in until your spine is almost perpendicular to the floor. As you exhale, lift your legs, keeping your knees bent. Slowly lift your knees up toward the ceiling as you bring your feet to the wall. Straighten your legs and rest your heels and buttocks against the wall.

Roll your thighs in, lift your tailbone, lengthen your legs upward, and keep your feet together. Balance on the crown of your head, press your forearms into the floor, and continue to lift your shoulders away from your ears. Keep your breathing even, your eyes and throat soft, and your abdomen relaxed. With regular practice, you can learn to bring your buttocks and heels away from the wall. Hold the pose as long as you can, up to 5 minutes.

To come out, exhale and bring your legs down to the floor one at a time. Bend your knees, sit back on your heels, with your head down, and rest for a few breaths before raising your head.

EFFECTS Like all inversions, this pose balances your neuroendocrine system. In particular, it stimulates the blood flow to your brain, activates your pituitary gland and pineal body, and energizes your entire body. Many women find Headstand (Sirsasana) beneficial when their depression is part of premenstrual or perimenopausal symptoms.

†CAUTION Do this pose only if it is already part of your yoga practice. Do not do this pose if you have high blood pressure, are menstruating, or suffer from neck or back problems or migraines. Instead move on to Wide-Angle Standing Forward Bend (Prasarita Padottanasana) on page 40.

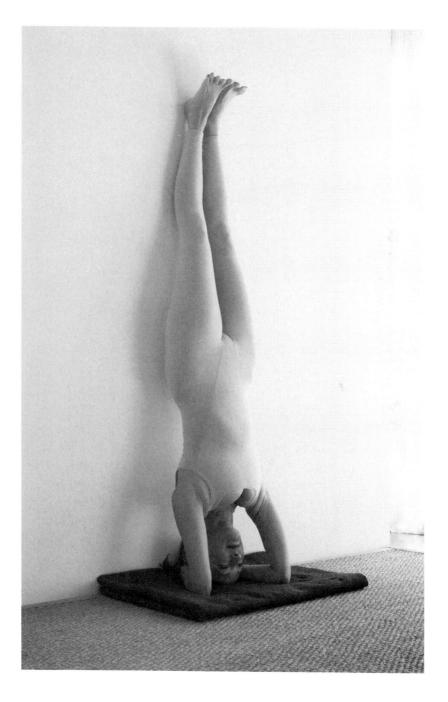

ALTERNATIVE: WIDE-ANGLE STANDING FORWARD BEND (Prasarita Padot-tanasana) If you don't practice Headstand (Sirsana), do this pose instead. Place two folded blankets or a bolster vertically in front of you. Step your feet wide apart (about 4 feet or so), keeping the outer edges of your feet parallel. Tighten your quadriceps to draw your kneecaps up and keep your thighs well lifted. On an exhalation, bend forward from your hips and place your hands on the floor between your feet. Lift your hips toward the ceiling; draw your shoulder blades into your back. Look up and extend your trunk forward, arching your back slightly. Remain this way for 5 to 10 seconds.

ALTERNATIVE TO HEADSTAND

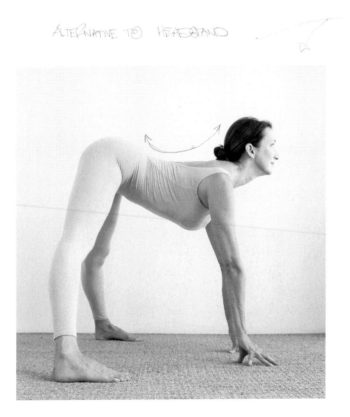

Keeping your trunk extended, exhale, bend your elbows, and release the crown of your head onto your support. Keep your legs firm, but relax your shoulders and neck. Breathe deeply and let your trunk release downward. Stay in this pose for 1 minute.

To come out, return to the concave back position, bring your hands to your hips, and raise your trunk. Step your feet together.

EFFECTS This pose is excellent for calming anxiety, jittery nerves, and mental or physical tension, as well as for combating fatigue.

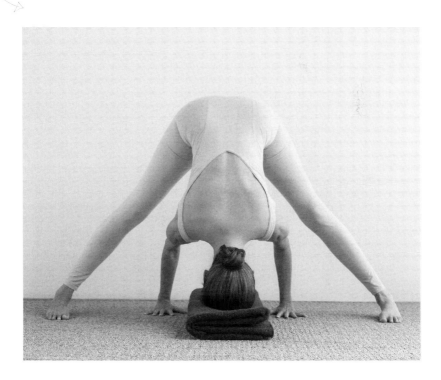

5. CAMEL POSE† **(Ustrasana)** Kneel on the floor with your knees and feet hip-width apart. Place your palms on your buttocks and as you exhale, move your thighs forward slightly and raise your side ribs. Gradually bend back as far as possible, lift your chest, and broaden your shoulders. Move your hands from your buttocks to your feet, and take hold of your heels. (If you can't reach your heels, place your hands on a chair positioned behind you, fingers pointing away from your body as much as possible.) Your thighs should be perpendicular to the floor. Take your head back, if that's comfortable, and breathe steadily for 10 to 15 seconds. If that's too difficult at first, come into and out of the pose a couple of times.

To come out, release your hands one at a time. As you exhale, slowly lift up from your sternum, using your thigh muscles. Your head should come up last.

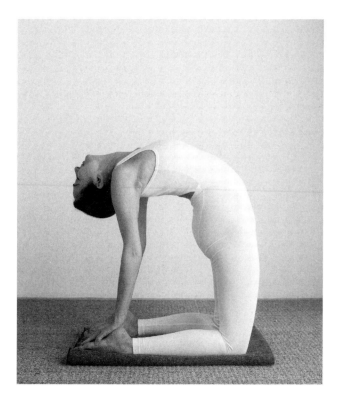

EFFECTS This pose opens your chest and brings energy, joy, and a sense of accomplishment. It has the added benefits of stimulating your vertebrae to retain calcium and building a strong spine and upper back muscles.

†CAUTION Do not do this pose if you have a migraine or tension headache, or if you suffer from hypertension.

MODIFICATION Position a chair so that the chair seat is closest to you. Kneel in front of the chair and rest your palms on the seat. Gradually arch your back and broaden your chest as you slide your palms toward the back edges of the chair seat. Take your head back, as long as you don't feel any tension or strain in the neck or throat. Press your shins and the tops of your feet into the floor and push your thighbones forward, away from the chair. Move your shoulder blades into the back ribs and roll your shoulders back. Remain in this pose, breathing evenly, for 20 to 30 seconds (or as long as 1 to 2 minutes). To come out of the pose, walk your hands toward the front edge of the chair seat as you lift yourself up. Use your thigh muscles and your chest to help move out of the back bend.

EFFECTS This pose is good for increasing lung capacity, increasing circulation throughout your body, and strengthening your back muscles. It will improve your posture, which can take pressure off your spine, and removes stiffness in the shoulders, knees, and ankles.

†CAUTION Do not do this pose if you have a migraine or tension headache, arthritis of the knees, or if you suffer from hypertension.

Modification

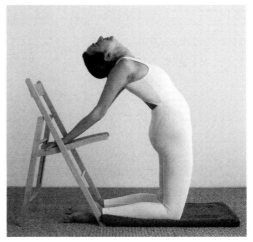

6. DOWNWARD-FACING DOG POSE (Adho Mukha Svanasana) Lie facedown on your sticky mat. Place your palms on the floor by each side of your chest with your fingers well spread and pointing straight ahead. Come up on your hands and knees. That's your position. Return to your hands-and-knees position and turn your toes under.

Exhale, press your hands firmly into the mat and extend up through your inner arms. As you exhale, raise your buttocks high into the air and move your thighs up and back. Keep stretching through your legs and bring your heels toward the floor. Keep your legs firm and your elbows straight as you lift your buttocks upward and release your head onto your support. The action of the arms and legs serves to elongate your spine and release your head. Hold this pose for 30 seconds to 1 minute, breathing deeply. Let your head rest completely and release the base of your neck. To come out, return to your hands and knees and sit back on your heels.

EFFECTS This is a wonderful pose to combat depression because it helps increase circulation to your chest, improve respiration, and calm your brain. This is a good counterpose to do after backbends. It stretches and tones your spine and releases tension in the back, neck, and shoulder areas. It further helps to combat depression by increasing circulation to your chest.

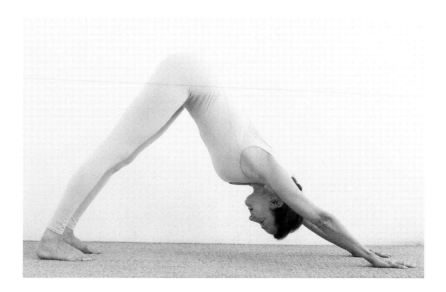

ALTERNATIVE: CHILD'S POSE (Adho Mukha Virasana) If Downward-Facing Dog (Adho Mukha Svanasana) creates strain or discomfort in your neck or shoulders (or lower back), practice this active child's pose instead. Kneel on the floor with your knees slightly wider than your hips and bring your big toes together. Bend forward and stretch your arms and trunk forward. Rest your head on the floor or a blanket. Remain in this pose for 20 to 30 seconds, moving your shoulder blades into your back ribs and elongating the back of your neck. To come up, press your hands into the floor and slowly sit up, lifting your head up last.

EFFECTS This pose stretches your back after backbends and helps calm your nerves.

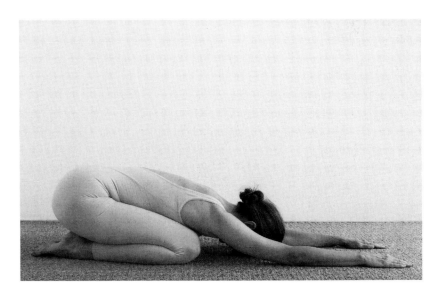

7. SHOULDERSTAND† **(Sarvangasana)** Place a chair with its back about 8 to 10 inches away from the wall. Put a folded sticky mat or blanket on the chair seat and two or three folded blankets in front of the chair. Sit backward on the chair with your legs bent over the top of the back; move your buttocks into the center of the chair seat (A).

Holding the sides and then the front legs of the chair, slowly lower your torso so your shoulders are on the blankets and your head is on the floor (B). You must extend your spine and open your chest while doing this to get the proper position. Move your hands, one at a time, to hold the back legs of the chair; your arms should be between the front legs. Stretch your legs out and rotate your thighs in (C).

†CAUTION Do not do this pose if you suffer from neck or shoulder problems, if you have high blood pressure, are menstruating, or if you have a migraine or tension headache.

A

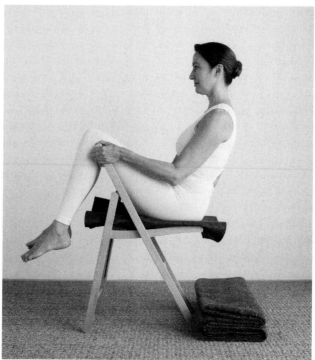

B

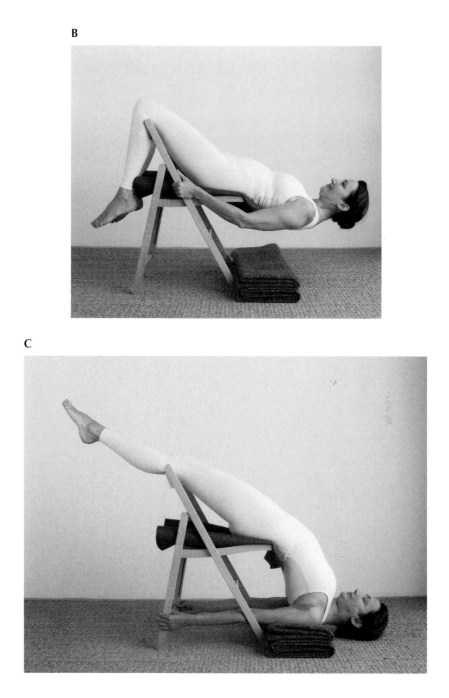

C

Lift your legs straight up (D) or rest your heels against the wall. Keep your legs together and extend from your groin to your heels. Close your eyes, bring your chest toward your chin, breathe normally, and hold for 3 to 5 minutes, or as long as you are comfortable.

D

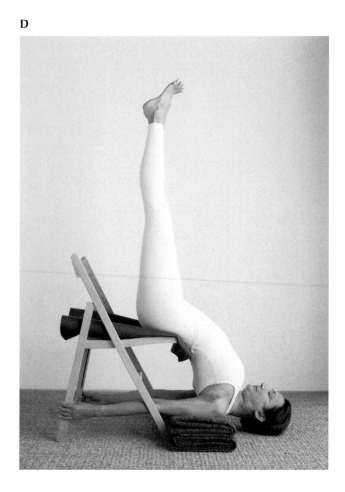

To release from the pose, bend your knees, place your feet on the chair seat (E), release your hands, and slide down until your sacrum rests on the blankets and your calves are on the chair seat. Rest on the floor a moment, then roll to your side and sit up slowly.

EFFECTS Sometimes called the "queen of all poses," this posture supplies fresh, oxygenated blood to your thyroid and parathyroid glands, stimulates the kidneys and adrenals, and soothes your nerves. It can also bring back peace and a new resolve when you feel tired, listless, or nervous.

ALTERNATIVE POSE: See **BRIDGE POSE** (Setu Bandha Sarvangasana) on page 51.

E

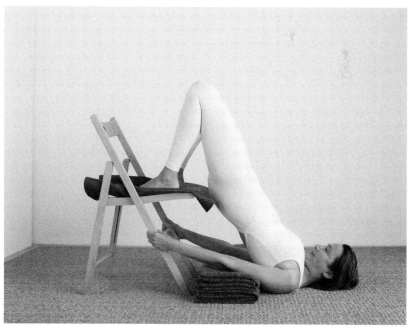

8. HALF-PLOUGH POSE† **(Ardha Halasana)** Place a folded blanket on your sticky mat with the rounded edge near the legs of a chair. Lie on your back with your legs outstretched, your shoulders on the blanket, and your head beneath the chair seat. As you exhale, bend your knees and swing or lift your buttocks and legs, so your thighs rest completely on the chair seat. (Pad the seat with blankets if you need more height for your legs to be parallel to the floor.) Move your chest in toward your chin (not your chin toward your chest). Relax with your palms up and your eyes closed. Remain in this position for at least 5 minutes.

To come out, place your hands on your back and slowly roll down, one vertebra at a time. Roll to one side and sit up.

EFFECTS Resting in this pose lifts your spirits and helps tame irritability and anxiety.

†CAUTION Do not do this pose if you suffer from neck or shoulder problems, or if you are menstruating.

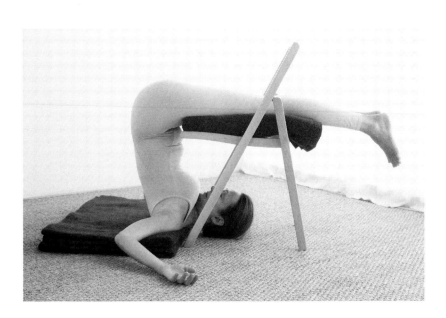

9. BRIDGE POSE (Setu Bandha Sarvangasana) Place a bolster horizontally against the wall and another vertically, forming a T shape. Place a folded blanket on the floor at the far end of the vertical bolster (for your head). Sit on the end of the vertical bolster that is closest to the wall. Keeping your knees bent, lie back over the bolster. Slide down until the end of the bolster is in the middle of your back and your shoulders just reach the floor. Rest your shoulders and head on the blanket. Stretch your legs toward the wall and put your heels on the horizontal bolster so your feet touch the wall. Your legs should be straight out in front of you, hip-distance apart. Rest your arms in any comfortable position. Close your eyes and relax completely, softening your abdomen and breathing deeply. Stay in this position for 5 to 10 minutes.

To come out, bend your knees and slowly roll to one side. Push yourself up to a seated position.

EFFECTS This pose opens your chest while bringing a sense of calm to your body and mind.

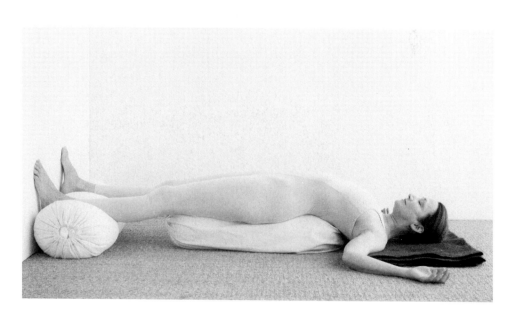

10. CORPSE POSE (Savasana) Lie on your back with your legs stretched out in front of you. Put a blanket under your head if you have tightness in your neck. Place your arms comfortably at your sides, slightly away from your torso, with your palms facing upward. Actively stretch your arms and legs away from you, then allow them to release completely. Close your eyes and let everything relax. Take a few deep breaths, inhaling into your chest without tensing your throat, neck, or diaphragm. Exhale your body into the floor, releasing your shoulders, neck, and facial muscles. Relax your pelvic floor muscle (the muscle you use to stop urinating) and the muscles in your buttocks and abdomen; release your lower back. As you relax, breathe normally for at least 10 minutes.

To come out of the pose, bend your knees, roll slowly to one side, and after a few breaths, gently push yourself to a seated position.

EFFECTS This is a very restful pose that can help you build confidence, relieve fatigue and depression, and rejuvenate your whole body. By helping to balance your sympathetic nervous system, it mitigates the effects of stress on your emotions as well as your body.

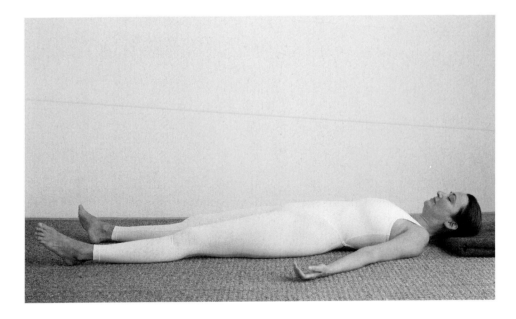

Chapter 4
The Lowdown on Low Bone Mass

IN ASSESSING YOUR RISK FACTORS, GENETIC OR OTHERWISE, YOU may be surprised to find that you fall into the high-risk category and you're a prime candidate for bone fractures. Convinced you have osteoporosis already (no matter what your age), you suddenly feel your bones aching and your upper back rounding. Is it really time to panic? Of course not. But today is as good a time as any to quit smoking; stop drinking coffee and soda; moderate your alcohol consumption; get a handle on your stress; and vow to give up your high-sugar, meat-at-every-meal diet plan. And either go back to or start doing yoga.

Determining the health of your bones (and whether you have osteoporosis right now) is difficult. Osteoporosis is known as a "silent" disease because most women don't know they have it until they break a bone. And low bone mass in itself does not automatically mean you have brittle bones or that you have a hip fracture waiting to happen. Only half of women with low-density bone mass experience a fracture; others with higher-than-normal bone density inexplicably break bones. Again, it's up to you to make sure the bones you have remain not only strong, but healthy and capable of repairing themselves.

If you're at high risk for osteoporosis and you've never had a bone mineral density (BMD) test, you may want to get one now, no matter how old you are, so you can establish a baseline reading. The most accurate test so far is the dual energy X-ray absorptometry (DEXA), and it's the one doctors prefer. This test measures your bone density and compares it to the bone density expected in someone your age. It also stacks your results against the "young normal," which means it compares your bones with those of someone at her peak bone mass (a thirty-year-old woman). Some doctors suggest you get several tests done over a twenty-four-month period so you can see how fast you're losing bone. But the prevailing wisdom at the moment is that these tests alone aren't good predictors of osteoporosis. Some doctors now recommend that you put off having a BMD test until you're at least sixty-five, unless you are at risk (see the list of risk factors on page 9). Another method of measuring possible bone loss is by a simple NTx urine test, which measures how much calcium is being excreted through your urine. A higher-than-normal reading may indicate that you are losing too much bone calcium.

REVERSING BONE LOSS

It's never too late to start taking care of your bones. Studies confirm that women who increase their mineral intake—calcium, magnesium, zinc, and potassium—improve their bone density. One such study published by M. Chapuy indicated that eighty-four-year-old women improved bone density in their hips by taking 1,200 mg/day of tricalcium phosphate and 800 IU of vitamin D. The control group, in contrast, lost bone density and had 67 percent more fractures. Preliminary research suggests that increased doses of vitamin D (upward of 3,000 IU/day instead of the recommended 800 IU) may actually reverse bone loss, especially when taken in combination with calcium and magnesium.

HOW YOGA CAN HELP

Yoga can help your bones gain density and resilience in several ways. In a 1988 article in *Yoga Journal*, Mary Schatz, M.D., says yoga can stimulate your bones to retain calcium, provided your body gets enough calcium in the first place. The secret? Yoga emphasizes weight-bearing

Patricia Says

- To keep joints mobile and flexible, move in and out of a pose several times before holding the position. Do not hold a pose too long or lock your joints, but focus on creating freedom in your joints.

- Don't practice poses that compress your spine—keep it elongated.

poses (like arm balances, inversions, and standing poses) that affect your whole body—spine, arms, shoulders, elbows, legs, knees, ankles, and feet—while encouraging full range of motion. In a small, as yet unpublished study conducted at California State University at Los Angeles in 2000, researchers discovered that yoga actually increases bone mineral density. Nine female subjects practiced yoga, and another nine did not. Researchers gave everyone bone density tests at the beginning of the study and again after six months. The yoga practitioners increased bone density in their vertebrae, but the nonpractitioners showed no change at all.

B. K. S. Iyengar contends that through the process of squeezing out the old, stale blood and lymphatic fluids, and soaking each area with freshly oxygenated blood or fluids, yoga helps your body use the nutrients it ingests, so that it doesn't need to leach minerals from your bones. Inversions, particularly Shoulderstand (Sarvangasana) and Plough Pose (Halasana), work particularly well. These poses, according to Iyengar, regulate your thyroid and parathyroid glands (critical for metabolism) by creating a chin lock that squeezes stale blood from your neck region. As you come out of the pose and release the lock, the area is bathed in fresh blood. In other words, inversions aid circulation in and around your head and neck, which can rejuvenate the glands. Inversions put a good deal of pressure on the neck and upper back, however, so individuals with brittle bones or vertebral fractures should avoid them.

In Patricia's practice, she teaches forward bends to quiet the adrenal glands, which mitigates the effects of cortisol on the body, and backbends to energize them. She says twists are also effective for regulating the adrenals so that those glands will provide adequate amounts of estrogen and androgen to keep bones healthy.

A consistent yoga practice can give you self-assurance and stability no matter what your age, but it can have a significant impact as you grow older. Many older people fall because they lose confidence in their ability to move properly; others suffer from weakened muscles (often from lack of use), poor posture, or arthritis. Yoga can help improve your posture and coordination, strengthen your muscles, increase your flexibility, and promote better balance.

The yoga poses in the following sequence are preventive in nature, but they have also been shown to reverse bone loss once it starts. You may do the full poses or practice the modifications and supported varieties, if those feel safer to you—you'll reap the same benefits.

A SEQUENCE FOR PREVENTING/REVERSING BONE LOSS

CAUTION Do not do this sequence if you already have osteoporosis or have suffered fractures in the past.

1. Wide-Angle Seated Pose I (Upavistha Konasana I)
2. Bound Angle Pose (Baddha Konasana)
3. Reclining Big Toe Pose I (Supta Padangusthasana I) to Reclining Big Toe Pose II (Supta Padangusthasana II)
4. Mountain Pose (Tadasana) with various arm positions
5. Standing Forward Bend (Uttanasana)
6. Downward-Facing Dog Pose (Adho Mukha Svanasana)
7. Extended Triangle Pose (Utthita Trikonasana)
8. Warrior II Pose (Virabhadrasana II)
9. Extended Side-Angle Pose (Utthita Parsvakonasana)
10. Warrior I Pose (Virabhadrasana I)
11. Intense Side Stretch Pose (Parsvottanasana)
12. Revolved Triangle Pose (Parivrtta Trikonasana)
13. Wide-Angle Standing Forward Bend (Prasarita Padottanasana)
14. Downward-Facing Dog Pose (Adho Mukha Svanasana)
15. Four-Limbed Stick Pose (Chaturanga Dandasana)
16. Upward-Facing Dog Pose (Urdhva Mukha Svanasana)
17. Camel Pose (Ustrasana)†
18. Upward-Facing Bow Pose (Urdhva Dhanurasana)
19. Child's Pose (Adho Mukha Virasana)
20. Bridge Pose (Setu Bandha Sarvangasana)
21. Legs-Up-the-Wall Pose and Cycle (Viparita Karani)†
22. Corpse Pose (Savasana)

†CAUTION You may want to skip or modify these poses due to health limitations or ability. Please read the explanatory footnote beneath the descriptions before giving them a try.

1. WIDE-ANGLE SEATED POSE I (Upavistha Konasana I) Sit on a block with your back against the wall and spread your legs wide apart; extend your ankles and spread and lengthen your toes. Adjust the flesh of your buttocks by drawing it behind you and out to the sides. Place your hands behind you on the block to help move your abdomen in and up, open up your chest more, and move your shoulder blades into your back ribs. Sit up tall, stretching from groin to heels and keeping your knees straight. Stay in this pose for 30 seconds or more, breathing normally.

EFFECTS This pose helps increase circulation to your pelvic region. It provides isometric weight-bearing benefits for hips, legs, and spine.

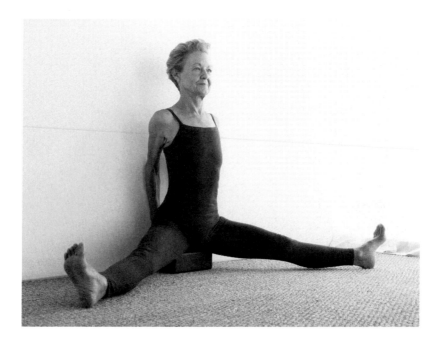

2. BOUND ANGLE POSE (Baddha Konasana) Sit on a block with your back against the wall and your abdomen lifted. Bending your legs, open your knees out to the sides and bring the soles of your feet together. Hold the tops of your feet and draw your heels in toward your pubic bone. The outer edges of your feet should remain on the floor. Place your hands on the block behind you. Lengthen your spine upward, leading with the crown of your head. (If you have trouble with this, place your hands on a chair in front of you for support.) Stretching your inner thighs from groin to knee, gently lower your knees as far as possible. Stay in this position for 30 seconds or more, breathing normally. To come out, relax your arms and bring your knees up one at a time.

EFFECTS The isometric stretch in this pose safely stresses the bones in the knees, feet, ankles, and hips. Sitting upright provides weight-bearing benefits to the sacrum and lumbar spine.

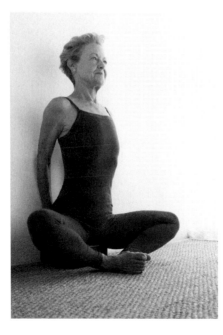

Modification

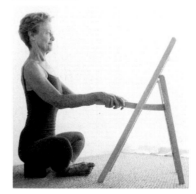

3. RECLINING BIG TOE POSE I (Supta Padangusthasana I) to RECLINING BIG TOE POSE II (Supta Padangusthasana II) Lie flat on the floor with your legs outstretched and together. As you inhale, draw your left knee up to your chest and place a strap around the ball of your foot. Exhale as you extend your leg straight up toward the ceiling (A). Hold the strap with both hands. Keeping your leg straight, move it closer to your head (if possible), and keep your pelvis firmly planted on the floor (B). Keep your right leg on the floor, actively pressing it into the ground, with your toes toward the ceiling. For additional support, press your foot into the wall. Move your leg gently back and forth in its socket to increase mobility and to keep the joints fluid. Move to the next pose before changing sides.

Keeping your left leg extended and your right leg on the floor, transfer the strap to your left hand and stretch your right arm out to the side. On an exhale, ease your left leg out to the side and down onto a bolster (C). Pull gently on the strap to add a little resistance. Rest comfortably for as long as you can, preferably 1 to 2 minutes. Repeat both poses with the right leg.

EFFECTS This active pose helps create more flexibility in your hip joints and groin, release stiffness in your lower back, stretch your hamstrings and calf muscles, and strengthen your knees.

A

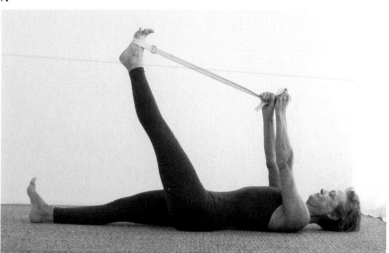

B

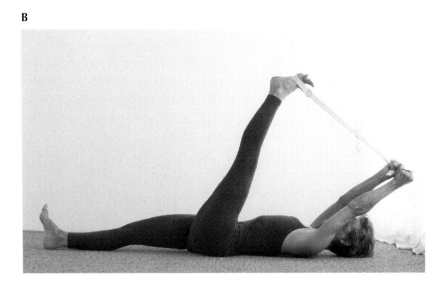

C

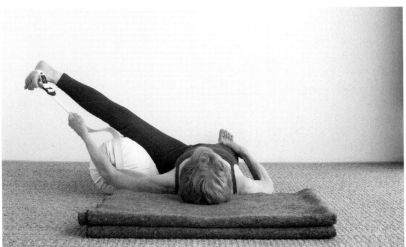

4. MOUNTAIN POSE (Tadasana) Stand up straight, your legs together. (Big toes should be touching, if that's comfortable. If not, hip-distance apart is fine.) Distribute your weight evenly between the front of your feet and your heels. Tighten your knees by pulling up with your quadriceps (front thigh muscles). Raise your sternum (breastbone) and broaden your chest by moving your shoulder blades into your back ribs. Move your abdomen in and up and draw your tailbone in without pushing your thighs forward. Extend your arms downward with palms facing your thighs and fingers together (A). Keep your shoulders moving away from your ears. It is normal to have some curvature in your lumbar area (lower back). Breathe normally, and gently lift from your pelvic floor muscles (the ones you contract to stop urinating). Continue to move your shoulder blades down into your back ribs, and elongate your neck. Remain in the pose for 30 to 60 seconds.

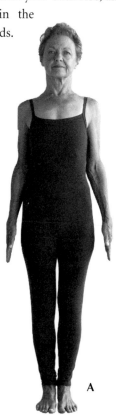

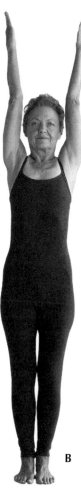

A   B

ARMS OVERHEAD (Urdhva Hastasana) Standing in Mountain Pose (Tadasana), turn your palms outward and slowly lift your arms to the side and over your head, keeping your shoulders down and away from your ears (B). Lift your chest and move your shoulder blades deep into your back ribs. (If you have trouble with balance, you may step your feet apart a little or practice with your back against a wall.) Stay in this pose for 20 to 30 seconds, if possible. Otherwise, come in and out two to three times. With your arms up, proceed to the next pose.

ARMS OVERHEAD WITH INTERLOCKING HANDS (Baddhangullyasana) With your arms overhead, bring your hands together, interlock your fingers, turn your palms toward the ceiling, and lengthen up through your inner arms. Move your shoulder blades into your back ribs, lift your sternum (breastbone), and stretch up through your side body. Hold this pose for 10 to 20 seconds and slowly release your arms down by your sides.

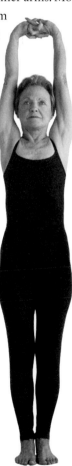

ARMS IN PRAYER POSITION (Namaskar) To further open your chest and shoulder area, continue standing in Mountain Pose (Tadasana). Take your arms behind your back and press the fingertips of both hands together with your fingers pointing down. Rotate both arms and wrists so that the fingers point in toward your back and then up. Keeping this arm position, slide your hands up your back, preferably all the way up so your hands are in line with your shoulder blades. Pressing your palms together evenly, keep your fingers extended. Rotate the shoulder bones back and move the shoulder blades into the back ribs. Your elbows should move toward the floor as you move your hands further up toward the back of your head. (C). (If this is too much of a stretch, simply cross your arms behind you, and hold on to your elbows.) Your posture should remain in alignment, just as it does when you have your arms by your sides. To come out of the pose, slide your hands down your back and return to Mountain Pose with your arms by your sides.

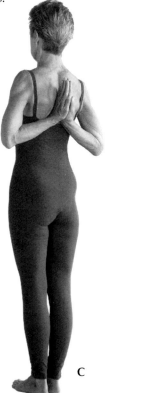

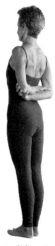

C   **Modification**

COW-FACE ARMS (Gomukhasana) Raise your right arm over your head, bend it at the elbow, and place the right palm, face down, just below the nape of your neck. Bend your left elbow, and raise your left forearm up behind your back, palm facing out, until your left hand is level with and between your shoulder blades. Clasp your hands behind your back or hold a strap if you can't catch your hands. Keep your right elbow pointing toward the ceiling and your head up. Roll your right shoulder back and bring your left armpit forward to open your chest. Be careful not to push your diaphragm and abdomen forward. Breathe normally in this pose for 30 seconds or more. To come out of the pose, unclasp your hands and bring your arms down by your sides. Repeat with your arms reversed.

EFFECTS The different arm positions help alleviate stiffness in your shoulders, arms, and upper and lower back; improve circulation throughout your body; and correct postural problems.

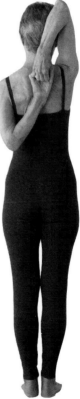

5. STANDING FORWARD BEND (Uttanasana) Balancing the weight evenly be-tween your feet, lengthen up through your inner thighs and roll your thighs in. Clasp your hands behind your back and keep your legs and knees firm as you stretch up through your waist and side ribs. On an exhale, lengthen your waist and side ribs toward the floor, bend forward, extend through your arms, and bring your hands overhead and down toward the floor. Keep your shoulders moving away from your neck and release your head down. Remain in this posi-tion for 10 to 15 seconds. To come out, release your hands, keep your legs active, and slowly lift to standing.

EFFECTS By clasping your hands behind your back, you open your chest more and release tension and stiffness in your shoulders, elbows, wrists, and fingers.

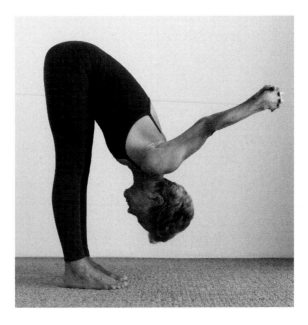

6. DOWNWARD-FACING DOG (Adho Mukha Svanasana) Place two blocks against the wall, shoulder-width apart. Kneel in front of the wall and place your palms on the blocks. Curl your toes under and walk your feet back, keeping them hip-width apart, so they are about 4 feet away from and in line with your hands. Keeping your hands on the blocks, lengthen up through your inner arms, and as you exhale, raise your buttocks high in the air. Stay on the balls of your feet as you move your thighs up and back. Keep stretching through your legs and bring your heels toward the floor. Keep your legs firm and your elbows straight as you lift your buttocks upward and release the crown of your head toward the floor. The action of the arms and legs serves to elongate your spine and release your neck and head. Hold this pose for 30 seconds to 1 minute, breathing deeply.

Come back to the hands-and-knees position. Bring your feet together, keep your knees slightly spread, and sit back on your heels. Bend down and rest your forehead on your mat. Let your arms lie by your sides with your palms up, and relax completely. Stay like this for a few full breaths.

EFFECTS This pose can brings weight-bearing benefits to your elbows, shoulders, wrists, and hands, as well as feet, ankles, knees, and spine. It also helps release stiffness in your back and hamstrings.

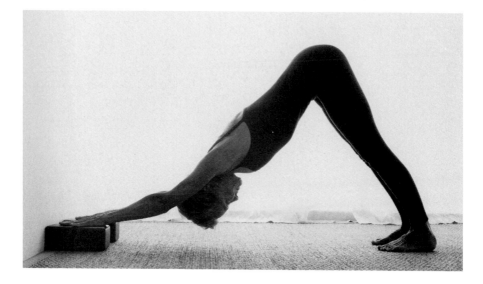

7. EXTENDED TRIANGLE POSE (Utthita Trikonasana) Stand in Mountain Pose (Tadasana). Step your feet about 3½ feet apart; turn your right foot out 90 degrees and your left foot slightly inward. The heel of your right foot should line up with the arch of your left. Place a block beside the outside edge of your right foot. Stretch your arms out to the sides, draw up through your quadriceps, and lift your abdomen and chest. On an exhalation, keeping your back straight, extend your trunk to the right and bring your right hand down to the block. Press your hand into the block, lengthen your spine, and expand your chest and

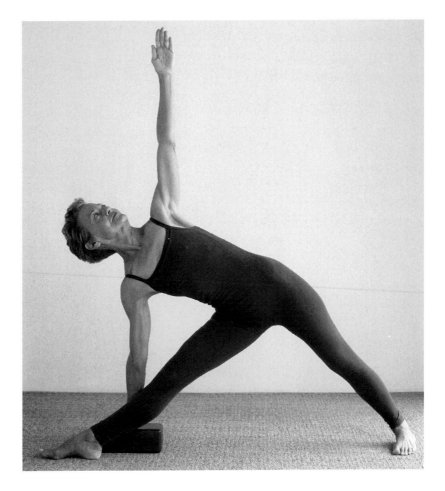

stretch your left arm up toward the ceiling. Draw your shoulder blades in, turn your chest and abdomen toward the ceiling, and look straight ahead or up at your left hand. Turn your abdomen to the left. Breathe normally and hold this pose for 20 to 30 seconds. To come out, press down through the left heel and inhale as you stretch up through the right arm. On an inhalation, lift up and straighten your torso. Repeat the pose on your left side, then turn your toes forward and step your feet back toward each other, returning to Mountain Pose.

MODIFICATION If this pose proves too challenging or if you feel unsteady, substitute a low stool or chair for the block. Place one hand on the chair and another on your hip. Keep your arms and legs active and strong. Move your shoulder blades into your back ribs. Relax your eyes, neck, and facial muscles, and breathe normally for several breaths.

EFFECTS This pose elongates and strengthens your spine and broadens the pelvis. It is excellent for helping increase flexibility and stability. Because it is a weight-bearing exercise for your arms, legs, pelvis, and spine, it stimulates the bones in those areas to retain calcium.

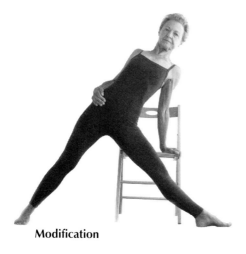

Modification

8. WARRIOR II POSE (Virabhadrasana II) Stand in Mountain Pose (Tadasana). Step your feet out as wide as possible (about 4½ feet apart, if you can); turn your left foot out 90 degrees and your right foot slightly inward. The heel of your left foot should line up with the arch of your right. Stretch your arms out to the sides so they're parallel to the floor. As you exhale, bend your left knee so your thigh is parallel and your shin is perpendicular to the floor. (If your knee extends beyond your ankle, you need to widen your stance.) Lengthen your spine, lift and extend your chest, and look over your left arm just past your fingertips. Extend the arms from the center of the chest out to the fingertips, as though your arms were engaged in a tug of war. If you can't hold this pose for more than 10 to 15 seconds, then move into and out of it two or three times. To

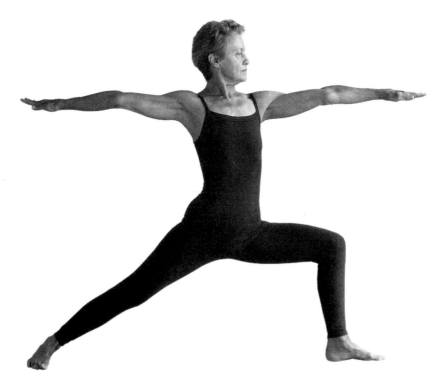

come out, straighten your left leg, press down through your left heel, and as you inhale extend up through your right arm. Repeat on the other side before stepping your feet together in Mountain Pose (Tadasana).

MODIFICATION If you need support, practice with one foot pressed up against and your hand resting on the wall (A). Move in and out of the pose by straightening as you inhale and bend the knee of the leg closest to the wall as you exhale, releasing your arms slightly, if necessary (B). This action will help to increase mobility in your joints. As you come into the pose for the last time, remove your hand from the wall, and remain in the pose for several breaths. Step your feet together and change sides.

EFFECTS This pose is great for improving posture, elongating and strengthening your spine, expanding your chest, and increasing flexibility and strength in your hips, back, and legs. Because it is a weight-bearing exercise for your feet, ankles, and legs, it stimulates the bones in those areas to retain calcium.

Modification A

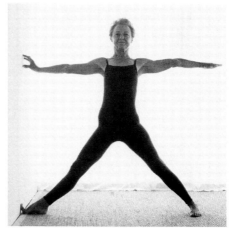

Modification B

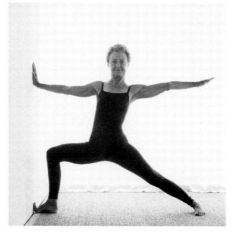

9. EXTENDED SIDE-ANGLE POSE (Utthita Parsvakonasana) Stand in Mountain Pose (Tadasana). Step your feet out as wide as possible (about 4½ feet apart, if you can); turn your left foot out 90 degrees and your right foot slightly inward. The heel of your left foot should line up with the arch of your right. Stretch your arms out to the sides. As you exhale, bend your left knee so your thigh is parallel and your shin is perpendicular to the floor. (If your knee extends beyond your ankle, widen your stance.) Keeping your back leg firm, exhale and lengthen out over your left thigh, bring your left hand down to the floor (or a block), and stretch your right arm up over your right ear. Move your shoulder blades into the back ribs, continue to lengthen your spine and turn your abdomen toward the ceiling, and look straight ahead or up toward the ceiling. Turn your abdomen to the right. Breathe normally and hold this pose for 20 to 30 seconds, if possible. To come out, straighten your left leg, press down through your left heel, and as you inhale, extend up through your right arm. Repeat on the other side before stepping your feet together in Mountain Pose.

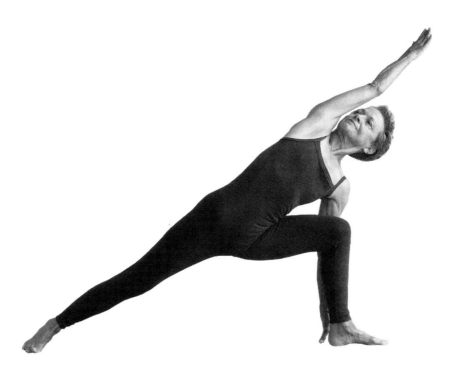

MODIFICATION If you need more support, rest your forearm on a chair positioned next to your bent leg instead of bringing your hand down to the floor or a block.

EFFECTS This pose broadens the abdomen, opens your hip joints, and elongates your spine. As a weight-bearing pose, it also helps strengthen your legs, knees, and ankles. It also relieves stiffness in your elbows, neck, and shoulders.

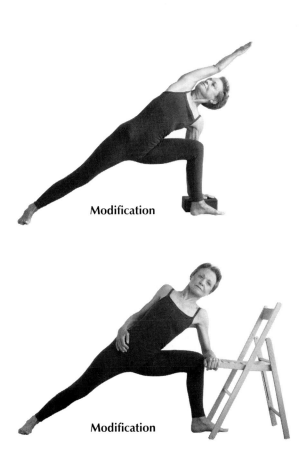

Modification

Modification

10. WARRIOR I POSE (Virabhadrasana I) Stand in Mountain Pose (Tadasana). Step your feet as far apart as is comfortable (about 4 to 4½ feet) with your toes pointing forward. Stretch your arms out to the sides at shoulder level, parallel to the floor, with palms down. Turn your palms up and stretch up through both arms until they are in line with your ears and parallel to each other; your elbows should be straight. Draw up through your quadriceps and lift your abdomen and chest. As you exhale, simultaneously turn your torso and right leg 90 degrees to the right and your left foot about 60 degrees to the right. Inhale and lengthen up through your upper arms; exhale and bend your right knee so your thigh and shin form a right angle. (If your knee extends beyond your ankle, widen your stance.) Keep a powerful extension of your back leg. Elongate your thoracic spine toward the ceiling. Keeping your sternum (breastbone) lifted, lengthen your neck, take your head back as far as it is comfortable, and look up toward your thumbs. If this is too hard on your neck, keep your head straight and your gaze soft. If you can't stay in the pose for more than 10 seconds, put your hands on your hips and move into and out of the pose several times to create mobility in your hips and knees.

MODIFICATION If you need additional support or stability, press the toes of your front foot into a wall and place your hands on the wall (A). Look straight ahead. Move in and out of the pose with each exhalation, keeping your back leg firmly extended and bending and straightening your front leg three or four times (B). As you bend your knee the last time, release your hands from the wall, and stretch your arms over your head with your palms facing each other. Keep your shoulder blades in and down, and open your chest. Remember not to let your knee extend beyond your ankle. Breathe normally for several breaths. Return to Mountain Pose (Tadasana) and switch legs.

EFFECTS This weight-bearing pose helps increase mobility in your hips and lower back. Moving in and out of the pose helps keep your joints flexible. This pose is a wonderful preparation for backbends and is particularly powerful for opening up the upper back and creating mobility in the shoulders. It increases flexibility in the thoracic spine and helps to move it into the chest and the chest up to the ceiling. Excellent for those with a curvature in the upper back (kyphosis or hyperkyphosis).

Modification A

Modification B

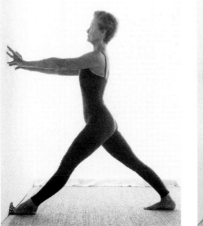

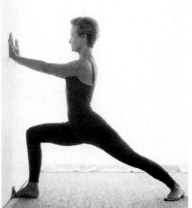

11. INTENSE SIDE STRETCH POSE (Parsvottanasana) Stand in Mountain Pose (Tadasana). Join your palms in prayer position behind your back. Roll your shoulders back and press your palms together to open your chest. (If this is too difficult, simply fold your arms behind your back, fingertips touching your elbows, or raise your arms over your head.) Raise your sternum. Step your feet about 3 to 3½ feet apart, so your weight is distributed equally between your legs. Turn your left foot 90 degrees and your right foot about 75 degrees to the

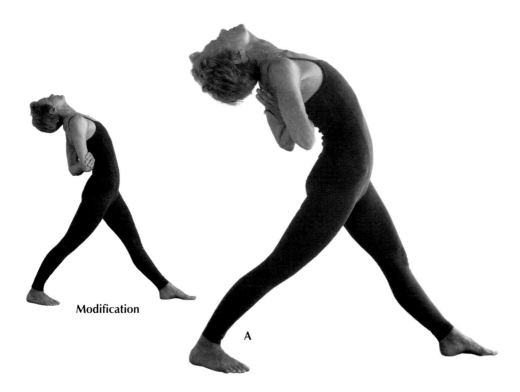

Modification

A

left. Turn your torso to face left, elongate the spine, lift the chest up toward the ceiling, and look up slightly (if that is comfortable on your neck) (A). Stay in this position for a few breaths. As you exhale, lower your chin and relax the abdomen and spinal muscles. Bend forward with your neck and spine in one plane as you lengthen your side body and release your head down toward your left shin (B). Keep both legs straight throughout the pose. Remain like this for 15 to 20 seconds, breathing normally. (If you have trouble balancing, put your hands on the floor, on blocks, or on your leg below the knee.) To come out, press down through your left heel, raise your head and torso together, and return to a standing position. Step your feet back together. Release your arms to the sides, return to center and repeat the pose on the other side.

EFFECTS This pose is especially beneficial for your upper back and relieves stiffness in your neck, shoulders, elbows, and wrists and helps ease the pain of arthritis, scoliosis, and kyphosis.

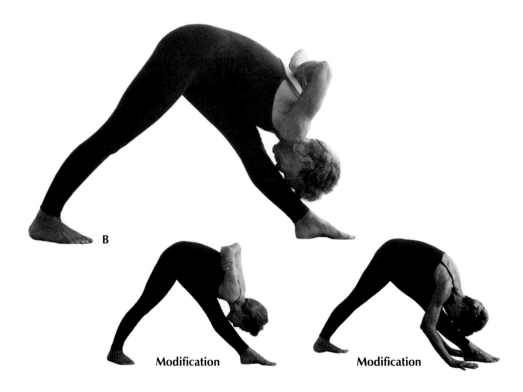

B

Modification   Modification

12. REVOLVED TRIANGLE POSE (Parivrtta Trikonasana) Stand in Mountain Pose (Tadasana). Step your feet about 3 to 3½ feet apart; turn your left foot out 90 degrees and your right foot slightly inward. The heel of your left foot should line up with the arch of your right. Place a block parallel to the outside edge of your left foot. As you exhale, rotate your torso so you are facing left; your right leg and knee should turn inward. Place the fingertips of your right hand on the block. Tighten both legs and keep your chest lifted and expanded by moving your shoulder blades into your back ribs. Breathe normally for 15 to 20 seconds. To come out, press down through your right heel, and as you inhale extend up through your left arm. Lift up slowly, straightening your torso. Repeat on the other side before stepping your feet together in Mountain Pose.

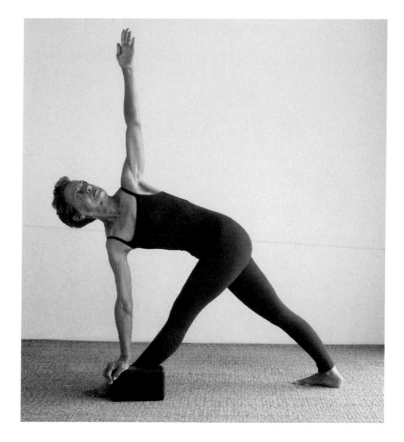

MODIFICATION If this pose is too difficult, place your forearm on a chair instead of a block. Add blankets and bolsters to the chair to raise the height, if necessary. Come in and out of the pose several times to keep your joints fluid and flexible. Hold the final pose for several breaths, if possible.

EFFECTS The weight-bearing action of this pose stimulates the bones in your legs, arms, and spine to retain calcium. It also elongates and strengthens your thoracic spine; increases flexibility and mobility in your shoulders, hips, and back; and improves your posture.

Modification

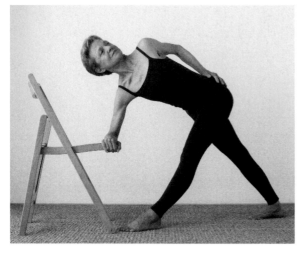

13. WIDE-ANGLE STANDING FORWARD BEND (Prasarita Padottanasana) Place two blocks, shoulder-width apart, in front of you on the floor. Step your feet apart about 4 feet (or as wide as possible), keeping the outer edges of your feet parallel. Tighten your quadriceps to draw your kneecaps up and keep your thighs well lifted. On an exhalation, bend forward from your hips and place your hands on the blocks underneath your shoulders and straighten your arms. Lift your hips toward the ceiling, move your inner back thighs away from each other as your lengthen your spine forward (toward your head). Move your upper spine in toward your chest. Move your shoulder blades into the back ribs

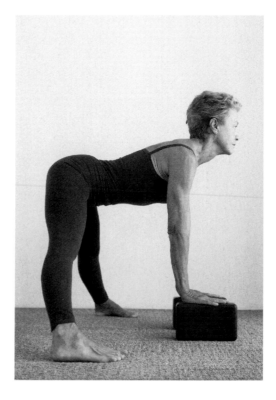

and look up. Your mid- to upper-thoracic spine will be slightly concave. Stay in this pose for 1 minute, if possible. Then release your head down, and place your hands on the floor, if possible. (If not, keep them on the blocks.)

To come out, bring your hands to your hips, raise your trunk, and step your feet together.

EFFECTS This position, especially the first part when your back is slightly concave and your head is up, lengthens your spine and moves it into alignment. This pose counters the forward curvature of the upper back and neck, especially for those suffering from kyphosis or hyperkyphosis.

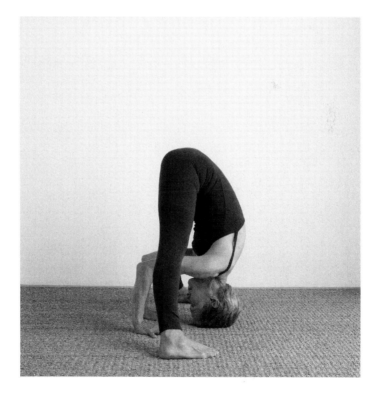

14. DOWNWARD-FACING DOG POSE (Adho Mukha Svanasana) Repeat Downward-Facing Dog Pose, without using the blocks at the wall. Begin on your hands and knees. Turn your toes under and as you exhale, press your hands firmly into the mat and extend up through your inner arms. Exhale again, raising your buttocks high into the air and moving your thighs up and back. Keep stretching through your legs and bring your heels toward the floor. Keep your legs firm and your elbows straight as you lift your buttocks upward and release the crown of your head toward the floor. The action of your arms and legs serves to elongate your spine and release your head. Hold this pose for 30 seconds to 1 minute, breathing deeply. Either come back to the hands-and-knees position and sit back on your heels for a few breaths or move directly into the next pose.

EFFECTS This excellent all-around weight-bearing pose can help ease arthritic pain in your elbows, shoulders, wrists, and hands. It also helps release stiffness in your back and hamstrings.

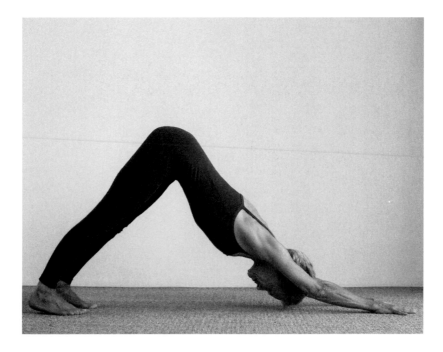

15. FOUR-LIMBED STICK POSE (Chaturanga Dandasana) Lying face down on the floor, bend your elbows and place your palms by your sides in line with the floating ribs. Your feet should be hip-distance apart and the toes anchored so that they point toward your head. Exhale and raise the entire body a few inches above the floor. (Alternately, you can begin the pose from Downward-Facing Dog Pose, coming forward so that your wrists are in line with your shoulders. Exhale as you slowly lower your body until it hovers a few inches off the floor.) Keep the chest, hips, thighs, and knees lifted so the whole body rests only on the hands and toes. The whole body and legs should be firm, like a staff and your face and chest should be parallel to the floor. To come out of the pose, exhale and lower your body down to the floor and rest for several breaths.

MODIFICATION If you have trouble pushing up or lowering down into the pose without collapsing in the shoulders or lower back, place a low block at your navel before you begin your push-up.

EFFECTS This yoga push-up stimulates the bones to retain calcium, and strengthens the muscles, in the shoulders, wrists, and elbows, as well as the legs, ankles, and knees. It builds strength, balance, and determination. Many women find it an exhilarating, confidence-inspiring pose.

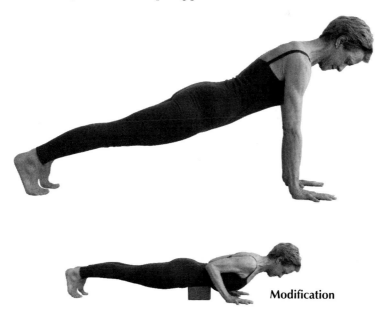

Modification

16. UPWARD-FACING DOG POSE (Urdhva Mukha Svanasana) Lie facedown with your feet about hip-width apart, your toes pointing back, and your legs active. Bend your elbows, spread your fingers, and place your palms on the floor by the sides of your chest. On an inhalation, raise your head and chest up, straightening your arms and elbows. Lift your pelvis, thighs, and knees away from the floor. Your weight should rest on your palms and the tops of your feet. Keeping your elbows straight, roll the shoulder bones back and lift the chest further. As you lengthen your neck, take your head back and look up. (If you feel discomfort in your neck, simply look straight ahead.) Remain in this position for 15 to 20 seconds. (Put your hands on blocks if you can't lift your thighs off the floor or open your chest.) To come out, exhale as you bend your elbows, resting the hips, thighs, and chest on the mat. Lower your head down and relax.

EFFECTS This pose is especially good for sciatica pain, stiffness in your shoulders and upper back, and lower back tension. Opening your chest can lift your spirits when you are depressed and help calm agitated or nervous energy.

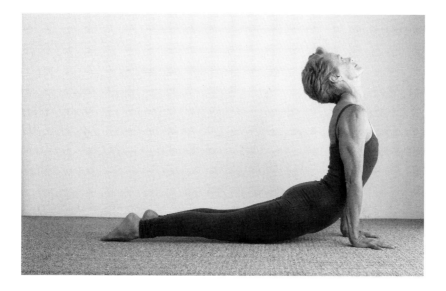

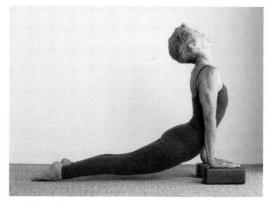

Modification

17. CAMEL POSE† **(Ustrasana)** Kneel on the floor with your knees and feet hip-width apart. Place your palms on your buttocks and as you exhale, move your thighs slightly forward and raise your side ribs. Gradually bend back as far as possible, lift your chest, and broaden your shoulders. Move your hands from your buttocks to your feet, and take hold of your heels. (If you can't reach your heels, place your hands on a chair positioned behind you.) Your thighs should be perpendicular to the floor. Take your head back, if that's comfortable, and breathe steadily for 10 to 15 seconds, if you can. To come out, release your hands one at a time. As you exhale, slowly lift up from your sternum, using your thigh muscles. Your head should come up last.

EFFECTS This pose brings weight-bearing benefits to the knees, ankles, and feet and is good for increasing circulation throughout your body and strengthening your back muscles.

†CAUTION Do not do this pose if you have a migraine or tension headache, or if you suffer from hypertension.

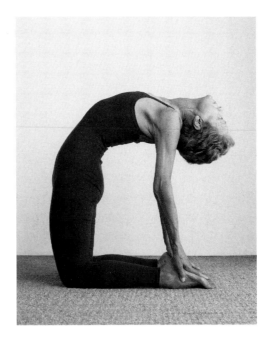

MODIFICATION Position a chair so that the chair seat is closest to you. Kneel in front of the chair and rest your palms on the seat. Gradually arch your back and broaden your chest as you slide your palms toward the back edges of the chair seat. Take your head back, as long as you don't feel any tension or strain in the neck or throat. Press your shins and the tops of your feet into the floor and push your thighbones forward, away from the chair. Move your shoulder blades into the back ribs and roll your shoulders back. Remain in this pose, breathing evenly, for 20 to 30 seconds (or as long as 1 to 2 minutes). To come out of the pose, walk your hands toward the front edge of the chair seat as you lift yourself up. Use your thigh muscles and your chest to help move out of the back bend.

EFFECTS This pose is good for increasing lung capacity, increasing circulation throughout your body, and strengthening your back muscles. It will improve your posture, which can take pressure off your spine, and removes stiffness in the shoulders, knees, and ankles.

†CAUTION Do not do this pose if you have a migraine or tension headache, arthritis of the knees, or if you suffer from hypertension.

Modification

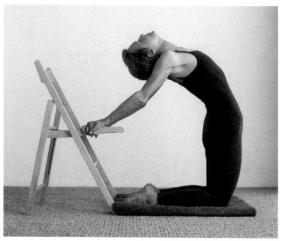

18. UPWARD-FACING BOW POSE† (Urdhva Dhanurasana) Lie on your back with your knees bent, your feet hip-width apart, and your heels close to your buttocks. Bend your elbows and place your hands alongside your head with your fingers pointing toward your feet. As you exhale, raise your hips and chest, straighten your arms, and stretch your legs. Lift your tailbone and move the backs of your thighs and your buttocks up toward the ceiling. To come out of the pose, bend your knees and elbows, and slowly lower your body to the floor. Hold this pose for 5 to 10 seconds, if you can. If not, come in and out of the pose two or three times.

MODIFICATION If you have trouble pushing up into a backbend, try this pose with blocks and a bolster. Position two blocks against the wall, shoulder-width apart, with a vertical bolster between them, touching the wall (A). Lie on your back on the bolster, with your head closest to the wall. Bend your elbows and place your hands on the blocks, fingers pointing toward your feet. Push up as instructed above (B).

EFFECTS This pose improves circulation throughout your body, stimulates your entire nervous system, expands and opens the chest, and generates an overall feeling of elation and well-being.

†CAUTION Do the unsupported version of this pose only if it is already part of your yoga practice. Seek the advice of an experienced teacher if you have neck problems. Do not do this pose if you have a migraine or tension headache, suffer from high blood pressure, neck or shoulder problems, or any serious illness, or are pregnant.

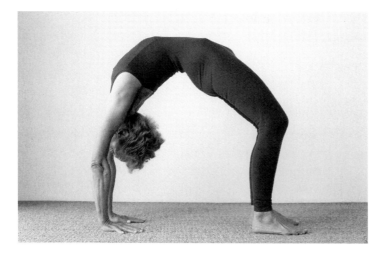

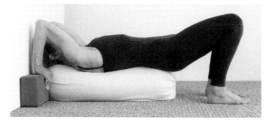

Modification A

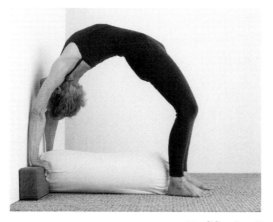

Modification B

19. CHILD'S POSE (Adho Mukha Virasana) Kneel on the floor with your knees slightly wider than your hips and bring your big toes together. Bend forward and stretch your arms and trunk forward. Rest your head on the floor or a blanket. Remain in this pose for 20 to 30 seconds, moving your shoulder blades into your back ribs and elongating the back of your neck. To come up, press your hands into the floor and slowly sit up, lifting your head up last.

EFFECTS This pose stretches and tones your entire spine while releasing the muscles in your neck and upper back. This pose also stretches your back after backbends and helps calm your nerves.

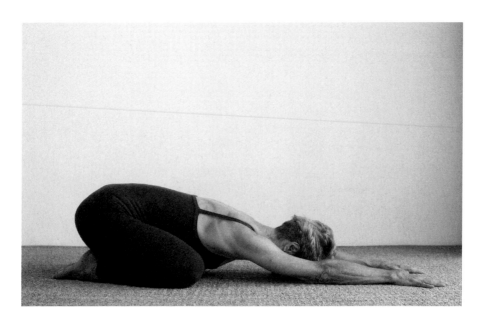

20. BRIDGE POSE (Setu Bandha Sarvangasana) Place a block vertically against the wall and have another at your side. Lie on your back with your arms at your sides and your knees bent. Place a blanket under your head to release the back of your neck, especially if you have rounding in the thoracic spine. Raise your hips and chest as high as possible and support your back with your hands, fingers pointing in toward your spine. Keeping your head and shoulders flat on the floor, lift your spine even farther, increasing the arch, and place the other vertical block under the fleshy part of your buttocks. Stretch out one leg at a time, resting each heel on the vertical block against the wall. Release your arms so that your hands reach just beyond the block. (If that is uncomfortable, bend your arms at right angles, fingers facing toward your head, and relax. See modification.) Hold the pose for at least 30 seconds, breathing normally.

To come out, bend your knees and place your feet on the floor. Then release the block under your sacrum and slowly roll down one vertebra at a time. Hug both knees to your chest and rest for several breaths.

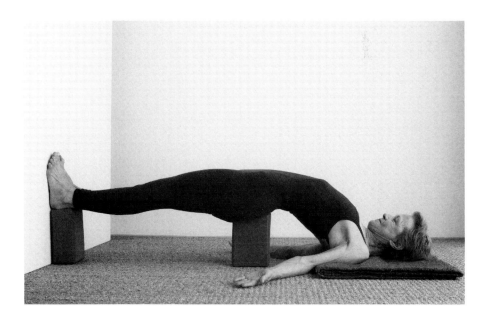

MODIFICATION Place a bolster horizontally against the wall and another verti-cally, forming a T shape. Fold a blanket on the floor at the far end of the vertical bolster for your head. Sit on the end of the vertical bolster that is closest to the wall. Keeping your knees bent, lie back over the bolster. Slide down until the end of the bolster is in the middle of your back and your shoulders just reach the floor. Rest your shoulders and head on the blanket. Keeping your feet and heels together, stretch your legs toward the wall and put your heels on the horizontal bolster so your feet touch the wall. Your legs should be straight out in front of you. Rest your arms in any comfortable position. Close your eyes and relax completely, softening your abdomen and breathing deeply. Stay in this position for 5 to 10 minutes.

To come out, bend your knees and slowly roll to one side. Push yourself up to a seated position.

EFFECTS Use this posture to help tone your kidneys and adrenal glands. This gentle backbend opens the back and releases the shoulders.

Modification

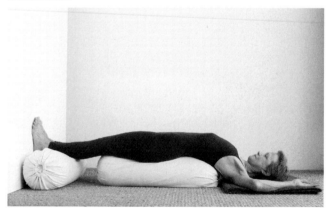

21. LEGS-UP-THE-WALL POSE AND CYCLE† (Viparita Karani) Place a bolster about 3 inches from the wall. (If you are tall, you may need a higher support, such as a folded blanket on top of the bolster.) Sit on the bolster so your right hip and side are touching the wall. Using your hands to support you, lean back and swivel your body around, taking your right leg and then your left leg up the wall. Keep your buttocks close to or against the wall. (If you feel stiffness or discomfort in your legs, push your buttocks slightly away from the wall.) Lie down so your lower back and ribs are supported by the bolster and your shoulders and head are on the floor. (If your neck is uncomfortable, put a rolled towel or blanket under it.) Extend through your legs and place your arms out at your sides, elbows bent and palms up (A). Rest in this position, eyes closed, for at least 5 to 10 minutes.

†CAUTION Do not do this pose if you are menstruating.

A

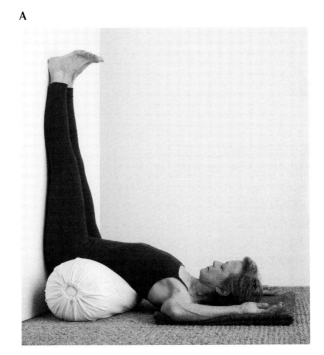

CYCLE Without moving your torso, allow your legs to open out to the sides (B). Remain in this position, breathing normally, for 3 to 5 minutes.

Again keeping your torso in the same position, bend your knees, cross your legs and the ankles, and continue in the pose for another 3 to 5 minutes (C).

To come out, bend your legs, rest the soles of your feet against the wall, and gently push away from the wall until your buttocks are off the bolster and resting on the floor (D). Roll to one side. Breathe quietly for a few breaths, then use your arms to help you to a seated position.

EFFECTS This pose relieves nervous exhaustion and helps balance your nervous system, mitigating the effects of stress hormones (cortisol and adrenaline).

B

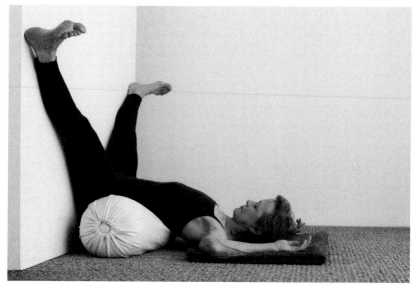

C

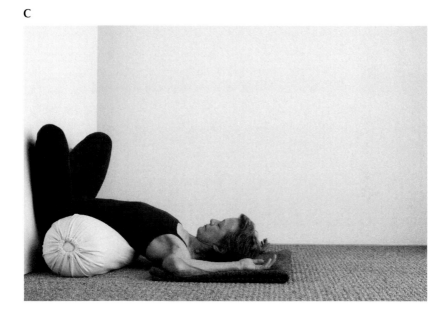

D

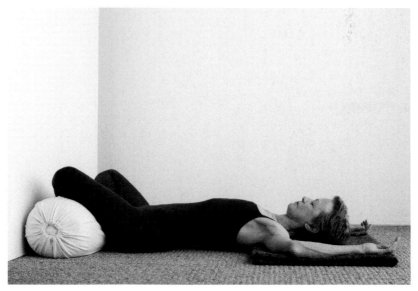

22. CORPSE POSE (Savasana) Lie on your back with your legs stretched out in front of you and your head comfortably supported. Place your arms by your sides, slightly away from your torso, with your palms facing upward. Actively stretch your arms and legs away from you, then allow them to release completely. Close your eyes and let everything relax. Take a few deep breaths, inhaling into your chest without tensing your throat, neck, or diaphragm. Exhale your body into the floor, releasing your shoulders, neck, and facial muscles. Relax your pelvic floor muscle (the muscle you use to stop urinating) and the muscles in your buttocks and abdomen; release your lower back. As you relax, breathe normally for at least 10 minutes.

To come out of the pose, bend your knees, roll slowly to one side, and after a few breaths, gently push yourself to a seated position.

EFFECTS This is a very restful pose that can help your body integrate the effects of your yoga practice. It builds confidence, relieves fatigue and depression, and rejuvenates your whole body.

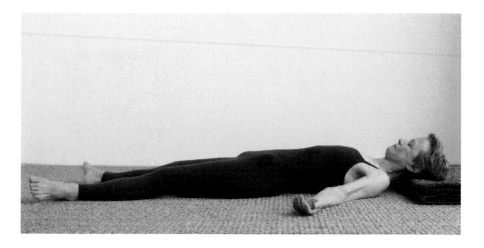

Moving Along Poses

Full-Arm Balance (Adho Mukha Vrksasana): Full Arm Balance, if it is already part of your practice, is a wonderful weight-bearing pose that builds not only stronger bones, but self-confidence as well.

Stand in Mountain Pose (Tadasana) facing a wall. Bend forward and place your hands, fingers spread, shoulder-distance apart, about a foot away from a wall. Keep your arms fully stretched and your shoulder blades moving into your back ribs. Take your legs back and bend your knees. Exhale and kick your legs up, one at a time if necessary, until they rest against the wall. Drop your head down and remain in the pose for up to one minute, if possible. If your hands are too far away from the wall, the curvature of your spine will be too great, and you'll feel strain in your lower back. Once you can balance with your feet on the wall, try moving them off the wall; then stretch your legs fully and point your toes toward the ceiling. To come out of the pose, rest your legs back on the wall, and slowly bring one leg at a time down to the floor. Sit back into Child's Pose for a few breaths before sitting up.

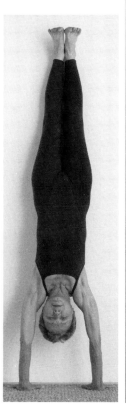

Caution Do not do this pose if you have problems with your wrists or shoulders, or if you are menstruating.

Chapter 5
The Osteoporosis Diagnosis

IF YOU'VE BEEN DIAGNOSED WITH OSTEOPOROSIS OR HAVE LOST A significant amount of bone mineral density, check with your health practitioner before you begin any yoga program. You may not even be aware that you've broken any bones, but if you've lost at least two inches in height, chances are you've already experienced vertebral fractures. An X ray can determine that.

Having osteoporosis presents sufferers with a classic catch-22. If you do too much exercise—or the wrong kind—not only will you be in pain, you may well break more bones. But if you don't exercise, your muscles will grow stiffer and weaker, and you'll lose the vital calcium and other minerals you need to prevent additional fractures. A diagnosis of osteoporosis is no longer an automatic death sentence; it can be a reversible condition. But to avoid future fractures and to increase bone density, flexibility, and strength, you need to be mindful of how you treat your body: give it the right kind of exercise, feed it properly, and maintain a positive outlook. It's imperative that you seek advice from a therapeutic yoga teacher and a knowledgeable health practitioner to create the right balance of activity and rest and to develop a sound diet that will support the health of your bones.

POOR BALANCE

To add insult to injury, older women who have osteoporosis tend to fall more often than their strong-boned counterparts. Failing eyesight, forward head position, weak muscles, and a large dose of insecurity or fear increase the likelihood of falling down; brittle bones almost ensure that they will break something when they do fall. According to Mary Schatz, M.D., in a *Yoga Journal* article, a lack of exercise affects coordination just as much as it does muscle tone, so older, less active women tend not to catch themselves when they start to fall. According to Schatz, "Neuromuscular coordination is also affected by posture. Information about the position of the head is sent to the brain from the joints between the cervical vertebrae. In older people with forward head carriage, this feedback system becomes faulty." In other words, when they stumble, this faulty feedback system prevents them from being able to recover their balance. Every slip becomes a potential disaster.

HYPERKYPHOSIS

Although kyphosis, or rounding of the upper thoracic spine, is listed as a significant risk factor for osteoporosis, having kyphosis does not mean you have osteoporosis. Only half of the women suffering from this condition experience fractures, and in those who do, the fractures generally occur first, causing the back to round. According to Gail Greendale, M.D., a gerontologist at the University of California, Los Angeles (UCLA), 30 percent of vertebral fractures are symptomatic (painful). As a woman bends forward to escape the pain, she puts more pressure on the anterior (front) part of her spine and suffers more fractures, creating a domino effect. In the other half of hyperkyphosis sufferers, the condition may simply result from poor alignment. Bad posture, a weak shoulder girdle, forward head position, flexed hips, and bent knees all contribute to what Dr. Greendale calls the "kyphotic posture." So, if we postulate that kyphosis is part posture and part structural curvature in the bone itself, those who have it can at least improve the posture element through yoga. No amount of yoga will straighten bone, however.

KYPHOSIS

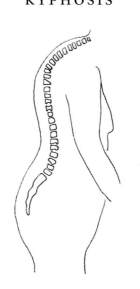

Annie Carpenter, a long-time yoga teacher from Yoga Works in Santa Monica, California, believes kyphosis punishes women in more than just physical ways. In her work with hyperkyphotic women, Annie has often seen the emotional repercussions of this condition. She observes that as the curve in the upper back becomes more pronounced the abdomen tends to protrude more and breathing becomes more labored and shallow. Many of the women she has spoken with express frustration and embarrassment about their bellies, so much so that they stop eating and going out. They don't exercise much either, because they can't breathe fully enough. As a result, they become oxygen starved, movement starved, depressed, and lonely. And because they don't eat well, they typically don't take in enough vitamins and minerals for their bodies to be fully alive and healthy.

HOW YOGA CAN HELP

Yoga is wonderfully adaptable. When you're healthy and strong (and have no symptoms), you can do yoga unsupported and take your body

Patricia Says

If you already have osteoporotic fractures, follow these tips:

- Avoid sudden or jerky movements.
- Do not do Headstand (Sirsasana) or other unsupported inversions that could bring weight to bear on your spine.
- Do not do forward bends. They can compress the anterior (front part) of your spine and increase the likelihood of additional fractures.
- Do not do balancing poses without the support of a chair or wall.

through its full range of motion. You reap the full benefits of standing poses, inversions, backbends, forward bends, and twists. The weight-bearing poses strengthen your bones; others balance your nervous system and give you confidence; still others bring a deep sense of relaxation and joy. And when you have brittle bones or have experienced fractures, you can still do yoga and gain similar benefits, but you must modify your practice so it works for your body in its present condition.

In setting out to prove that yoga can have a positive affect on hyperkyphotic women, Dr. Greendale hypothesized that yoga could "improve physical and emotional functioning as well as combat some of the underlying muscular and biomechanical causes" of the condition. In 1999, she invited Carpenter to participate in a pilot research study to measure such affects on women in their sixties, seventies, and eighties. Carpenter, Dr. Greendale's own yoga teacher, designed and taught a highly modified practice for this fragile-boned group, emphasizing the breath and the *essence* of the classical asanas, since the "final," or full, poses would likely never be achieved or even attempted. Carpenter says, "The process of designing this practice became an inspirational investigation into the *intention* of the asana practice as opposed to the achievement of asana as an end in itself." In other words, could these women reap the benefits yoga has to offer by doing the smallest amount of movement possible? The findings appear to indicate that they could—and did. In the Greendale study, twenty-one women took Carpenter's one-hour yoga classes twice a week for twelve weeks. They also kept journals of their experiences, in which they responded to loosely structured questions and added comments of their own.

Dr. Greendale is quick to point out that this was only a pilot study, and as such, had no control group against which to compare results. The participants were handpicked and hand-taught, and each had at least a forty-degree thoracic curvature. Greendale and her team put the women through a number of tests to ensure that they could do the yoga classes safely; everyone was deemed physically able to participate, and Greendale felt they wouldn't push themselves to do more than they were capable of doing. The program centered around four yoga sequences, which Carpenter modified to accommodate the students' physical status. The poses targeted neck and shoulders, spinal erectors (the muscles that support the spine), and the abdominals—the joints and muscles most commonly associated with kyphosis. She introduced new, more challenging poses every three weeks.

Greendale's study measured several outcomes: height without shoes, distance from tragus (ear) to wall (when standing with back against the wall), and kyphotic angle (degree of thoracic curvature). She also measured certain physical performance criteria. For example, could the

Sylvia's Story

Sylvia Unger was one of the oldest participants in the Greendale study—eighty-six years old. Her doctor recommended she sign up because of her kyphosis, so she did. But she never imagined it would make her feel so good. She's always been a walker; she walked alone several miles a week until her recent fall. Now she walks with friends. She thinks yoga helped her recover more quickly and prevented her from breaking any bones. But the best part of doing yoga for Sylvia is the way it makes her feel (so much taller). She's not sure she's actually grown—she thinks she might have—but it doesn't matter. She feels taller. And now when she sees her reflection in shop windows, it makes her happy.

participants move from standing to a seated position more quickly than before taking yoga classes? Did their functional reach (arm extension) improve? Could they pass the "penny test" (picking up a penny from the floor) or the "book test" (putting a book up on a high shelf)?

The age of the participants ranged from sixty-three to eighty-six years. Nine of the women had no thoracic or lumbar fractures, seven had at least one thoracic fracture, and five had both thoracic and lumbar fractures. Overall, the results were quite promising: the height of the participants increased and the distance from tragus to wall decreased. All the timed tests (going from sitting to standing, the penny test, and the book test) showed faster results, and everyone's functional reach improved. The only thing that didn't improve was the kyphotic angle. But the women looked and felt different. As Dr. Greendale observed, "These women came into the study feeling their bodies had failed them." Their yoga practice helped them figure out a way to encourage their bodies to work for and not against them. Many of them came in angry and finished the program full of joy and a "playful reawakening." When Greendale observed the class in Corpse Pose (Savasana), she exclaimed, "They all looked like angels, and they looked 10 years younger."

TWO SEQUENCES FOR WOMEN WITH KYPHOSIS AND/OR SPINAL FRACTURES

The first of this chapter's sequences is designed to foster more upright posture and to improve strength and balance. Women who have kyphosis are more likely to have osteoporosis, which puts them at higher risk of bone fracture if they fall or apply too much pressure to their bones. In addition, these women have problems balancing, and they often suffer from muscle weakness or other medical conditions that may make doing yoga risky. This sequence is not intended for anyone who needs a cane or walker or who has fallen and sustained injuries. In order to do this sequence, make sure you are able to do the following:

- Stand up from a seated or prone position and go from standing back down to the floor smoothly and with good control.

- Lift your arms to at least shoulder height without losing balance.
- Stand with feet hip-width apart for at least one minute and maintain good balance.

Women who have any medical conditions or health problems should discuss their desire to do yoga with their health practitioner before beginning this series—or any other yoga sequence.

Remember, yoga should always feel good, both in the moment and afterward. While you may experience a small amount of muscle soreness the day after you practice, you should never feel any pain or excessive fatigue. Your breathing can clue you in on how you're doing. If you can remain calm and focused, and your breathing is smooth and steady throughout, you are probably enjoying a safe and beneficial yoga practice. If your breath becomes ragged or you find yourself holding your breath, you're probably doing too much. Only after you feel completely comfortable doing the first sequence should you move on to the second. Do each sequence slowly and with loving kindness toward your body.

A SEQUENCE FOR OSTEOPOROSIS OR KYPHOSIS

For women who have osteoporosis or kyphosis, this gentle, safe sequence will relax tension, encourage deeper breathing, open the chest, and build strength in the upper back. Any time you lie on your back, pad your head with one or more folded blankets so that your chin isn't pointing toward the ceiling and you're not compressing the back of your neck.

1. Corpse Pose (Savasana) with Three-Part Breathing (Pranayama)
2. Corpse Pose with Arms Overhead (Urdhva Hastasana in Savasana)
3. Shoulder Girdle Press
4. Pelvic Tilt (Setu Bandha Sarvangasana)
5. Locust Pose (Salabasana) with different arm positions
6. Twisted Stomach Pose (Jatara Parivartanasana)
7. Corpse Pose (Savasana)

1. CORPSE POSE (Savasana) Place two or more folded blankets on the floor to support your head and have a chair close by. Lie on your back, with the blankets under your head so that your forehead and chin are on a level plane. Rest your calves on the seat of the chair so that your thighs are nearly vertical. (If you are tall, you may need to put a folded blanket on the seat of the chair to raise your legs to the correct height.) Allow your head to rest completely on the blankets, and let your shoulders drop down toward the floor. Stay in this pose for at least 3 minutes before beginning the next pose.

EFFECTS This pose brings a sense of calm and serenity and puts you in touch with your breathing.

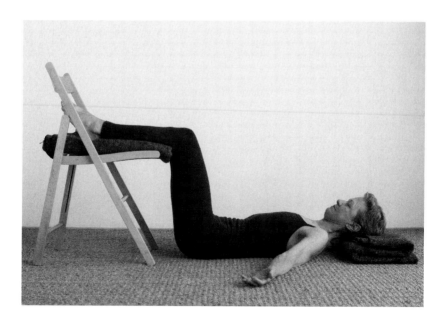

THREE-PART BREATHING (Pranayama) You may stay in the supported position on page 106, or lie on your mat with your legs outstretched, hip-width apart. Exhale completely. Inhale, focusing your breath into the lowest part of your ribs (floating ribs), expanding them sideways as well as front to back. Exhale completely. Inhale again into your floating ribs, then fill your middle ribs, again expanding fully, keeping your shoulders and neck soft. Exhale completely, first from your middle ribs and then from your lower ribs. Now inhale into your lower ribs, your middle ribs, and finally your upper ribs and the top of your chest, opening and expanding in all three directions (front, back, and sides). Very slowly exhale all the breath out of your body. Take a couple of easy breaths and repeat this cycle several times.

EFFECTS This simple pranayama sequence increases circulation in the lungs as well as the pelvis. Conscious breathing promotes a deep awareness of the whole body as it soothes and energizes simultaneously.

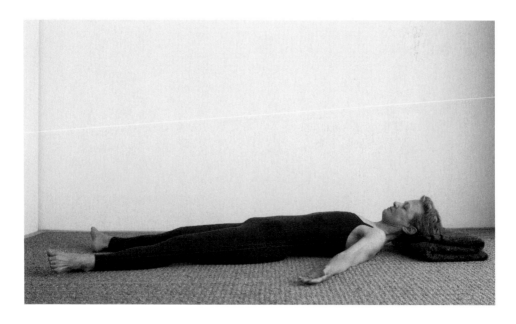

2. CORPSE POSE WITH ARMS OVERHEAD (Urdhva Hastasana in Savasana) Remaining in a supine position, bend your knees. Inhale and expand your chest. As you exhale, drop your shoulders down. Inhale as you lift your arms so that your fingers point straight up to the ceiling and your palms face each other. Exhaling, press your shoulders down to the floor and slide your shoulder blades down your back (A). Inhale and open your chest, then exhale as you lower your arms beside you. Repeat 5 times.

Inhale and expand your chest; as you exhale, drop your shoulders down. On your next inhalation, lift your arms so that your fingers point straight up and your palms face each other. As you exhale, press your shoulders into the floor and slide your shoulder blades down your back. Inhale and reach your arms over your head toward the floor, straightening them as much as possible when you exhale (B). Bring your arms to the floor if you can. Inhale and open your chest. Now exhale as you bring your arms back up over your head and lower your arms down to your sides again. Repeat 5 times. Rest.

EFFECTS This pose relieves stiffness in your shoulders, elbows, upper back, and neck.

A

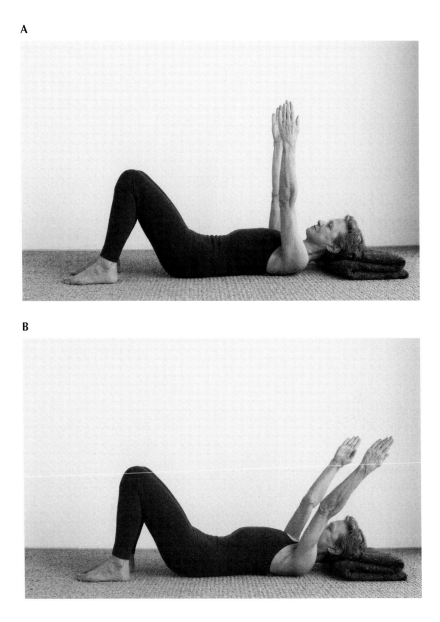

B

3. SHOULDER GIRDLE PRESS Remain on your back with your knees bent and feet flat on the floor, hip-distance apart. Inhale into your chest. As you exhale, press your shoulders and the backs of your arms into the floor. Inhale deeply again; exhale and relax. Repeat 5 times. Rest.

EFFECTS This pose releases your shoulder, neck, and pectoral muscles.

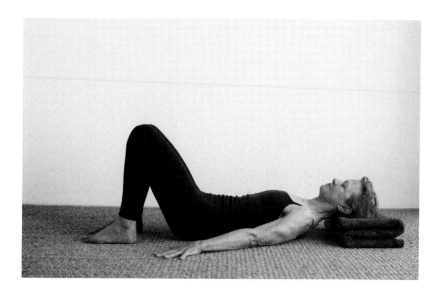

4. PELVIC TILT (Setu Bandha Sarvangasana) Inhale to expand your chest. As you exhale, lengthen your hips toward your heels. Inhale and press your feet into the floor; lift your hips off the floor. Make sure that your hips, knees, and ankles remain in line with one another. Exhale and release your hips down to the floor. Repeat 5 times. Rest.

EFFECTS This pose helps relieve stiffness in your sacrum and lumbar spine. It also brings weight-bearing benefits to your feet, ankles, knees, and hips.

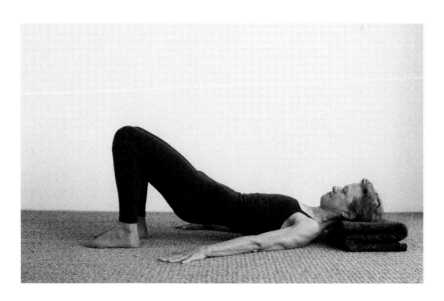

5. LOCUST POSE (Salabasana) Carefully turn over on your belly. Align your head with your spine, placing either your chin or your forehead on the floor. Extend your legs straight out behind you, making sure they are parallel. (If you feel any pressure in your lower back, you may place a folded blanket under your waist.)

CONTRALATERAL ARMS Extend both arms in front of you in a V shape so that your hands are a bit wider than shoulder-width. Turn your arms so that your palms face each other and your pinkies are on the floor. Inhaling, lift your right arm off the floor, reaching it as far forward as possible (A). Exhale as you slowly lower it again. Repeat with your left arm. Repeat this cycle 5 times.

Now, on an inhalation, lift your right leg up just a little, extending it back as much as you can, and then exhale as you slowly release it down. Repeat with your left leg and continue for 5 cycles. Rest.

Turn your palms down flat on the floor. As you inhale, lift your right arm and left leg as high as you can, keeping them as straight as possible, lengthening and extending them away from each other (B). Exhale and lower both limbs. Repeat with your left arm and right leg. Continue until you complete 5 cycles. Rest.

A

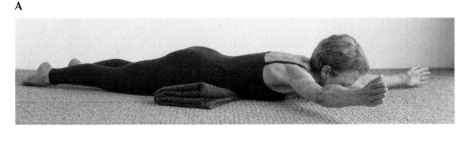

B

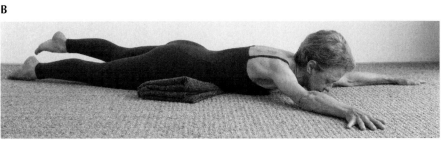

ARMS TO THE SIDES Stretch your arms straight out to the sides from your shoulders. Turn your arms so that your palms are facing forward. Inhale, lift your arms a few inches off the floor and stretch them out, away from you. Exhale and draw your shoulder blades down your back. As you inhale, lift your head, neck, and chest up (C)—any amount—and then exhale, slowly lowering everything back to the floor. Take a full, smooth breath. Now, inhale and extend both legs back and up—again, any amount (D). Exhale and lower them. Take another full breath. Repeat this cycle, first with your arms and chest, then with your legs, 5 times. Rest.

EFFECTS Locust Pose and all its variations relieve stiffness in the spine. It brings isometric weight-bearing benefits to the arms, shoulders, elbows, and spine.

C

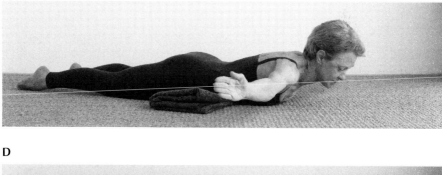

D

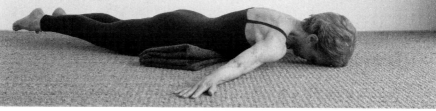

6. TWISTED STOMACH POSE (Jatara Parivartanasana) Lie on your back, knees bent and feet flat on the floor, hip-width apart. (Support your head with blankets if you need to.) Inhale and stretch your arms out to the sides at shoulder-height, with your palms facing up. Raise your feet slightly off the floor, and, exhaling, allow both knees to drop gently to the left until you feel a soft twist in your hips and low back. Take a few full breaths, and try turning your head and neck very slowly toward the right. Take a deep breath in, then on the exhalation, carefully bring your knees and head back to center. Take a full breath and repeat on the opposite side.

EFFECTS This is an important pose for building core strength, which is essential for balance and strength.

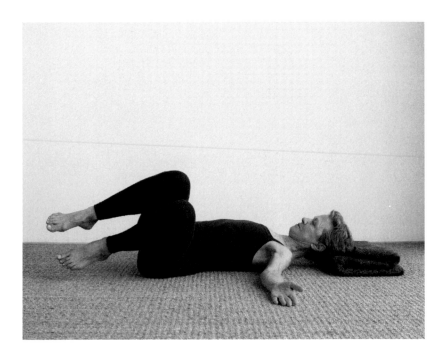

7. CORPSE POSE (Savasana) Place two or more folded blankets on the floor to support your head and have a chair close by. Lie on your back, with the blankets under your head so that your forehead and chin are on a level plane. Rest your calves on the seat of the chair so that your thighs are nearly vertical. (If you are tall, you may need to put a folded blanket on the seat of the chair to raise your legs to the correct height.) Allow your head to rest completely on the blankets, and let your shoulders drop down toward the floor. Stay in this pose for at least 3 minutes before beginning the next pose. Close your eyes and relax for 5 to 10 minutes.

EFFECTS This pose is not only profoundly relaxing and restorative, but it also integrates the effects of the whole previous sequence.

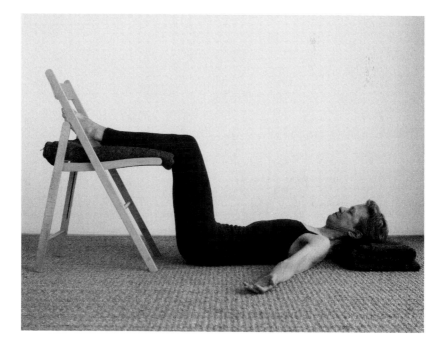

A CHAIR SEQUENCE FOR HYPERKYPHOSIS

1. Staff Pose (Dandasana) with Victorious Breathing (Ujjayi Pranayama)
2. Staff Pose with Arms Overhead (Urdhva Hastasana in Dandasana)
3. Staff Pose with Arms in Prayer Position (Namaskar in Dandasana)
4. Leg Raises (Utkatasana Prep)
5. Mountain Pose (Tadasana)
6. Mountain Pose with Arms Overhead (Urdhva Hastasana in Tadasana)
7. Fierce Pose (Utkatasana)
8. Warrior I Pose (Virabhadrasana I)
9. Half Downward-Facing Dog Pose (Ardha Adho Mukha Svanasana)
10. Simple Seated Twist Pose (Bharadvajasana)
11. Corpse Pose (Savasana)

This moving-along sequence is designed for women who can already do the floor sequence comfortably. Before you begin, make sure you are able to stand up from a seated position and then sit back down with relative ease. Use the chair as a prop in the standing poses to help you balance; go slowly and mindfully, using your breath to gauge your progress. This series of poses will strengthen your spinal erector muscles (those muscles that run alongside the spine); improve your posture, which will take pressure off your spine; and create better balance and more self-confidence. A combination of gentle weight-bearing poses and isometric movements will serve to build muscle and bone mass slowly and safely.

1. STAFF POSE (Dandasana) Sit forward far enough in a chair so that your back does not touch the back of the chair. Place your feet flat on the floor (put a pair of blocks under them if they don't reach comfortably), hip-width apart, with your toes pointing straight ahead. You can place your hands on the seat of the chair by your hips and press down through your hands to help you sit taller. Bring your pelvis to an upright position, and elongate your spine till you feel your head floating upward. Relax your face and gaze steadily at a single point directly in front of you. Gently roll your shoulders back and, as you deepen your breathing, allow your chest to lift and open.

EFFECTS This pose provides isometric weight-bearing benefits to the spine, sacrum, and shoulders.

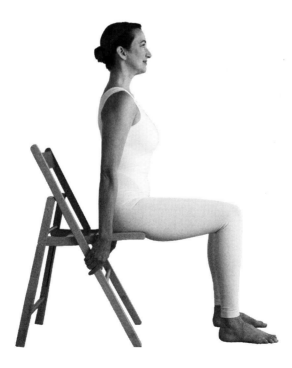

VICTORIOUS BREATHING (Ujjayi Pranayama) Remain sitting tall and observe your breathing. Exhale a long, slow breath. Inhale very slowly and deeply (without strain), expanding your lungs front and back, side to side, and up and down. Then exhale easily, keeping your chest lifted. Continue for 5 to 10 cycles, keeping your gaze steady and your face soft. Return to normal breathing.

Now, we'll concentrate on the exhalation. Exhale completely, and inhale easily. Exhale very slowly but without any strain. Try to be empty of breath before your next easy, steady inhalation. Repeat for 5 to 10 cycles, then return to normal breathing.

Now, exhale completely. Inhale slowly and fully, smoothly expanding your chest. Maintain the lift you have created in your chest and exhale slowly, fully, and smoothly. Connect the end of this exhalation seamlessly with the beginning of the next inhalation and the end of that inhalation with the following exhalation. Repeat for 5 to 10 cycles. Return to normal breathing.

EFFECTS If you have hyperkyphosis, you often have trouble breathing and getting enough oxygen into the lungs. Ujjayi Pranayama expands the lungs, soothes the nerves, and brings joy to the whole being.

2. STAFF POSE WITH ARMS OVERHEAD (Urdhva Hastasana in Dandasana) Sit forward and upright in your chair. Inhale, filling your chest. Exhale as you reach your arms straight down beside you. Inhale as you lift your arms forward so they are pointing straight out from your shoulders and your palms are facing each other. Exhale and draw your shoulder blades into your back. Inhale slowly and raise your arms as high as comfortably possible. Lower them as you exhale. Repeat 5 times.

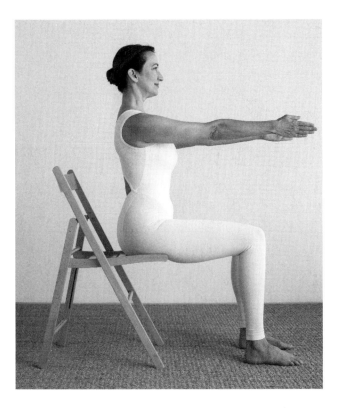

3. STAFF POSE WITH ARMS IN PRAYER POSITION (Namaskar in Dandasana)
Sit forward and upright in your chair. Bring your hands together in front of
your heart in prayer position. Inhale, expanding your chest. Exhale gently and
press your hands together, drawing your shoulders down and back while bringing your shoulder blades together and in (A). Inhale and open your bent arms
to the side, pressing with the entire back of your arm (B). Exhale and return to
the prayer position. Repeat the cycle 5 times.

EFFECTS This pose brings weight-bearing benefits to your upper body, most
particularly to your hands, arms, elbows, and shoulders. It also promotes core
abdominal strength.

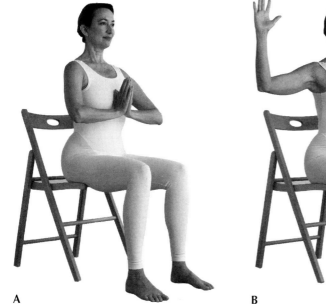
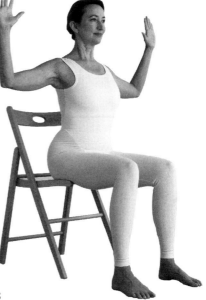

A   B

4. LEG RAISES (Utkatasana Prep) Sitting forward and upright on your chair, hold on to the seat or sides for balance. Inhale and lift your right foot off the floor, keeping your knee bent and your back as straight and upright as possible. Exhale and put your foot back on the floor. Change to your left leg; repeat 5 times.

Now, as you inhale, lift your right leg; extend out through your foot, straightening your leg as much as possible, as you exhale. Inhale and bend your knee, keeping your leg lifted. Exhale and return your foot to the floor. Switch legs. Repeat 5 times.

EFFECTS This pose promotes balance and core abdominal strength and relieves stiffness in the knees, legs, and hips.

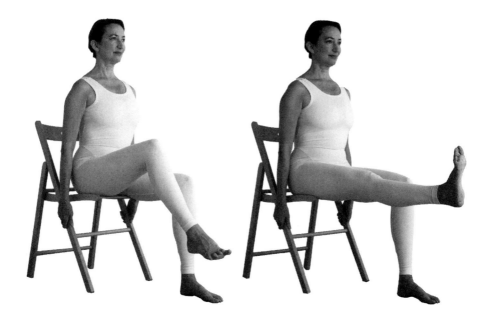

5. MOUNTAIN POSE (Tadasana) Stand tall with your feet hip-width apart, and have a chair just off to the side for balance. Take a full breath into your chest rolling your shoulders toward your back. Observe how you are balanced on your feet and see if you can spread your toes apart. Rock your weight back toward your heels and then forward toward your toes; sway back and forth a few times, gently and slowly, holding on to the chair with one hand, if you need to. Pay attention to what you need to maintain a sense of equilibrium. Bring yourself to a place that feels like center, and stand still and tall. Steady your gaze straight out in front of you and breathe deeply for a few cycles.

EFFECTS This pose promotes good posture, balance, and extends the spine. It brings weight-bearing benefits to the legs and feet.

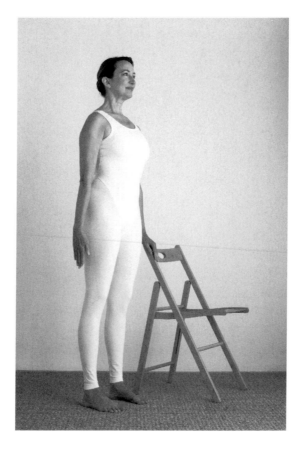

6. MOUNTAIN POSE WITH ARMS OVERHEAD (Urdhva Hastasana in Tadasana)
Still standing tall, feel your weight spread throughout your feet and breathe deeply into your chest. Hold on to the chair with one hand and as you inhale, lift your other arm out to the side. As you exhale, turn your extended arm from the shoulder so that your palm faces up. Inhale and reach your arm up as high as you comfortably can. Let go of the chair, if possible, and raise that arm up so it is parallel to the other. Stay for a breath or two. As you exhale, let both arms float slowly downward. Repeat 5 times. Rest.

> EFFECTS This is a wonderful pose for increasing self-confidence and improving balance.

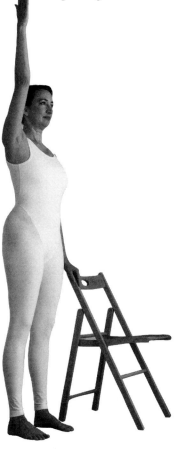

7. FIERCE POSE (Utkatasana) Stand tall with your feet hip-width apart and one hand on a chair beside you. Gently rock your weight toward your heels, and on an inhalation, slowly bend your knees as deeply as you can, keeping your heels down. Exhale and press your feet into the floor to straighten your legs and stand upright. Try to keep your torso upright as you bend each arm. Repeat 5 times. Rest.

Do the same pose again, with your free arm reaching up high as you bend your knees and coming down by your side as you straighten up. Repeat 5 times. Rest.

EFFECTS This pose strengthens your knees and legs and relieves stiffness in the legs and the lower back. It promotes good posture and increases core abdominal strength.

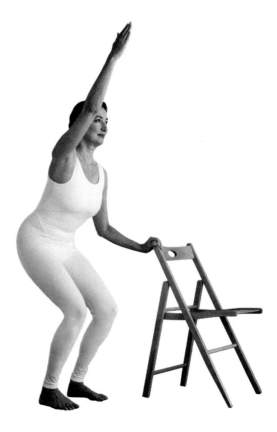

8. WARRIOR I POSE (Virabhadrasana I) Place your left hand on the back of the chair beside you. Step your right foot back about 2 feet or so, turning your toes slightly outward; keep your left foot facing straight ahead. Square your hips forward and firm your legs; inhale into your chest and stand as straight as you can. With your free hand on your hip, exhale and slowly bend your left knee so it points over your middle toe; try to keep your right foot flat. Inhale and slowly straighten your left leg, coming back to standing. Repeat 5 times, and work toward maintaining the squareness of your hips as you bend your leg. Move to the other side of the chair and repeat with legs reversed 5 times. Rest.

Going back to the first side, repeat the pose, this time lifting your right arm forward and up as you bend your left leg and inhale. Exhale as you straighten your leg and lower your arm. Repeat 5 times on each side. Rest.

EFFECTS This weight-bearing pose safely stresses the bones in the legs and feet. It increases mobility in the hips and lower back and helps keep your joints flexible. It also teaches you how to maintain better balance.

9. HALF DOWNWARD-FACING DOG POSE (Ardha Adho Mukha Svanasana)
Stand facing a wall and a few feet away from it. Your feet should be parallel and hip-width apart. Place your hands on the wall, leaning forward from your hips, not your waist. (If your legs feel tight or your back feels any strain, bend your knees a bit.) On an inhalation, press your hands into the wall with your fingers pointing upward, and squeeze your arms staight. As you exhale, reach your hips back away from your hands, stretching your spine. Take a breath or two. If this is fairly easy for you, try walking your hands down the wall, perhaps a few inches, and repeat the action of pressing your hands into the wall as you stretch back with your hips. Breathe here for a few breaths, if possible. Your hands may eventually line up with your hips so that your torso is parallel to the floor. Remember to work at your own pace and continue to breathe smoothly and fully. To come out of the pose, bend your elbows and walk your feet toward the wall. Stand still for a few breaths. Repeat the pose 5 times. Rest.

EFFECTS This pose brings weight-bearing benefits to the upper and lower body at the same time. It also relieves stiffness and tension in the upper back, neck, shoulders, wrists, and hamstrings.

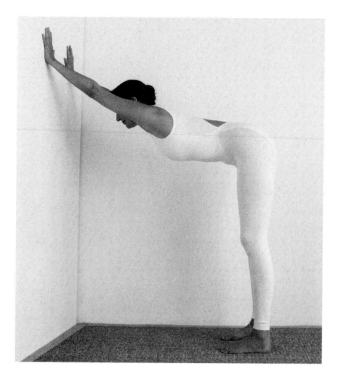

10. SIMPLE SEATED TWIST POSE (Bharadvajasana) Sit on your chair sideways (to the right), placing your feet flat on the floor so they're parallel and hip-width apart. Inhale and press gently down with your sitting bones and lengthen up through the crown of your head. Exhale as you start to twist, beginning with your waist and moving slowly upward to your ribs and chest. Place your left hand on your left knee, and try to put your right hand on the back of your chair. With each inhalation, stretch upward, and with each exhalation, gently twist a little more to the right. Perhaps eventually you can comfortably place both hands on the chair back. Keep releasing your shoulders back and down, so your chest is lifted and open. Take five or six breaths, then unwind slowly. Take a breath or two, and repeat on your left side.

EFFECTS This pose relieves stiffness in the spine and increases flexibility in the back. It also encourages core abdominal strength.

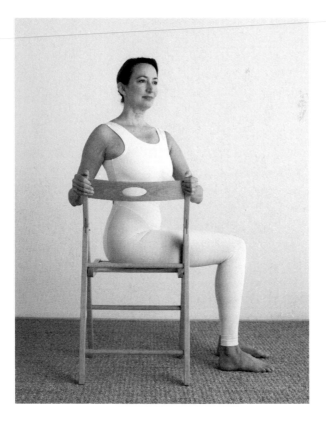

11. CORPSE POSE (Savasana) Place two or more folded blankets on the floor to support your head, and have a chair close by. Lie on your back, with the blankets under your head so that your forehead and chin are on a level plane, and rest your calves on the seat of the chair so that your thighs are nearly vertical. (If you are tall, you may need to put a folded blanket on the seat of the chair to raise your legs to the correct height.) Allow your head to rest on the blankets, and let your shoulders drop down toward the floor. Breathe normally and rest completely for at least 5 to 10 minutes. To come out of the pose, push yourself away from the chair with your feet, roll to one side, and use your arms to push yourself up.

EFFECTS This pose promotes deep relaxation as your body integrates the effects of your practice.

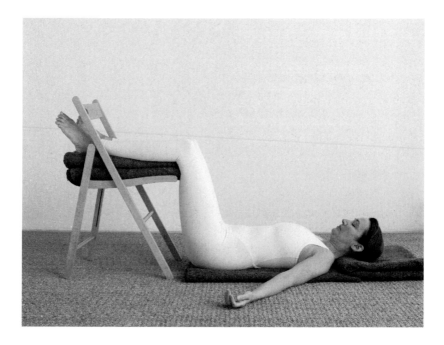

Chapter 6
Take Control of
Your Bone Health

READING THROUGH THIS BOOK YOU'VE LEARNED ABOUT THE various causes of osteoporosis and its sister condition, hyperkyphosis, and have no doubt come to realize that while this disease is largely caused by our Western lifestyle, it can also be prevented and/or remediated by changing that lifestyle. In this respect, it's much like type 2 diabetes: A percentage of those who suffer from osteoporosis have a genetic predisposition for the disease, but most bring it on through bad habits—poor nutrition, a lack of exercise, excessive consumption of alcohol, and smoking—and through an unrelenting amount of stress in their personal and professional affairs. All of these factors cause imbalances in the body or inhibit its ability to operate in the efficient manner nature devised. Thus, the body is forced to turn to the bones to supply its everyday need for calcium and other critical minerals—minerals the bones need to remain strong and resilient. Because we reach peak bone mass by our early thirties, most people use up the "dividends" that might provide calcium and end up living off their "principal deposit" (what's left in their bones). The financial analogy is especially apt, because in the end you're likely, quite literally, to go broke.

We've also talked a lot about how to live within your body's means by making a commitment to a healthy-bones regimen. It's time to stop talking about it and start taking action, no matter how old you are. If you're a mom, help your children make healthy-bone choices every day. Give them fruit and natural juices instead of colas or candy; feed them vegetables, whole grains, and seeds, and cut back significantly on the amount of meat they eat. Also, make sure they get ample amounts of potassium to mitigate the negative effects of that meat.

If you're a teenager, take control of your body now. Join a yoga class with a group of friends and make a commitment to one another to go at least three times a week. Learn how to prepare healthy snacks and meals for one another or for your family, that way you can help others benefit as well. Building up the health of your bones during your teens and twenties makes them less likely to suffer fractures when you get older.

Are you pregnant? Remember that strong bones begin in utero, so eat, breathe, and exercise for your baby's bones as well as your own.

And if, like many of us, you've reached a "certain age" without having taken care of yourself as well as you could have, don't despair. Despite the air of inevitability surrounding osteoporosis in the popular press, study after study has shown that a friendly bone regimen can improve bone mass and density even late in life. Start now. Quit smoking and cut back on or give up alcohol. Give your body the fuel it needs to maintain a healthy balance so it can stop borrowing minerals from your bones. That means changing your diet by adding lots of fresh green leafy vegetables and several daily servings of fruit, lentils, seed, nuts, and whole grains. Pick yourself up off the couch and get at least thirty minutes of weight-bearing exercise, especially yoga, every single day, so you can increase your muscle and bone strength and flexibility. And find ways to reduce the stress in your life—or at least learn how to control the way your mind and body react to today's stress-filled world. Do this not only for the health of your bones, but for every aspect of your physical, mental, and spiritual well-being.

Remember to laugh, spend time with people you love, and get outside to commune with nature. Meditate, read more, nurture yourself. How many times have you heard the phrase "your body is a temple"? It is indeed—one that requires a strong yet resilient foundation to support the vital, open, and loving self inside. Yoga can help you discover that self and give it the respect it deserves. Yoga will strengthen your bones in many ways, and just as important, it will also calm your mind and soothe your spirit. Remember, you deserve a strong, healthy, beautiful body; creating a healthy bone strategy is a great way to start.

Resources

I HAVE INCLUDED BOOKS, MAGAZINES, VIDEOS, INFORMATION SOURCES, and everything else I could think of in this list of resources that might help you on your journey toward wellness.

READING MATERIAL

This section includes the articles and publications mentioned in the book, as well as some others I think you may find useful.

Books

Brown, Susan. *Better Bones, Better Body: Beyond Estrogen and Calcium.* New York: McGraw Hill, 2002.

Fuchs, Nan Kathryn. *User's Guide to Calcium and Magnesium: Learn What You Need to Know about How These Nutrients Build Strong Bones.* North Bergen, N.J.: Basic Health Publications, 2002.

Gaby, Alan. *Preventing and Reversing Osteoporosis: What You Can Do about Bone Loss—A Leading Expert's Natural Approach to Increasing Bone Loss.* New York: Prima Publishing, 1995.

Gladstar, Rosemary. *Herbal Healing for Women: Simple Home Remedies for Women of All Ages.* New York: Simon & Schuster, 1993.

Hawkins, Steven, and Bea Beckman. *The Effect of Yoga on Bone Mineral Density and Body Composition in Adult Women.* Unpublished, 2000.

Iyengar, B. K. S. *Light on Yoga: Yoga Dipika.* New York: Schocken Books, 1979.

———, trans. *Seventy Glorious Years of Yogacharya.* Puna, India: Light on Yoga Trust, 1990.

Iyengar, Geeta. *Yoga: A Gem for Women.* Palo Alto, Calif.: Timeless Books, 1990.

Lonsdorf, Nancy, Veronica Butler, and Melanie Brown. *A Woman's Best Medicine: Health, Happiness, and Long Life through Ayurveda.* New York: Putnam, 1993.

Love, Susan. *Dr. Susan Love's Hormone Book: Making Informed Choices about Menopause.* New York: Random House, 1997.

Maddern, Jan. *Yoga Builds Bones: Easy, Gentle Stretches That Prevent Osteoporosis.* Gloucester, Mass.: Fair Winds Press, 2001.

Northrup, Christiane. *Women's Bodies, Women's Wisdom: Creating Physical and Emotional Health and Healing.* New York: Bantam Books, 1998.

Pert, Candace B. *Molecules of Emotion: Why You Feel the Way You Feel.* New York: Scribner, 1997.

Raman, Krishna. *A Matter of Health.* Madras, India: East-West Books, 1998. (Available through Iyengar yoga centers.)

Robertson, Joel C., with Tom Monte. *Natural Prozac: Learning to Release Your Body's Own Antidepressants.* New York: HarperCollins, 1997.

Scaravelli, Vanda. *Awakening the Spine: The Stress-Free New Yoga That Works the Body to Restore Health, Vitality, and Energy.* San Francisco: HarperSanFrancisco, 1991.

Schatz, Mary. *Back Care Basics: A Doctor's Gentle Program for Back and Neck Pain Relief.* Berkeley, Calif.: Rodmell Press, 1992.

Weed, Susun S. *Menopausal Years: The Wise Woman Way.* Woodstock, N.Y.: Ash Tree, 1992.

Woodman, Marion, with Jill Mellick. *Coming Home to Myself: Daily Reflections for a Woman's Body and Soul.* Berkeley, Calif.: Conari Press, 1998.

Journals, Magazines, and Newsletters

Canley, Jane, et al. "Effects of Hormone Replacement Therapy on Clinical Fractures and Height Loss: The Heart and Estrogen/Progestin

Replacement Study (HERS)." *American Journal of Medicine* 110, no. 6 (2001): 442–450.

Chapuy, M. "Vitamin D$_3$ and Calcium to Prevent Hip Fractures in Elderly Women." *New England Journal of Medicine* 327, no. 3 (Dec. 3, 1992): 1637–42.

Greenberg, R. P., R. F. Bornstein, M. J. Zborowski, S. Fisher, and M.D. Greenberg. "A Meta-analysis of Fluoxetine Outcome in the Treatment of Depression." *Journal of Nervous and Mental Diseases* 182, no. 10 (1994): 547–51.

Greendale, Gail A., Anna McDivit, Annie Carpenter, et al. "Yoga for Women with Hyperkyphosis: Results of a Pilot Study." *American Journal of Public Health* 92, no. 10 (2002): 1611–1614.

Schatz, Mary. "You Can Have Healthy Bones." *Yoga Journal.* (March/April 1988): 49–50.

Subscription Information

HerbalGram, P.O. Box 144345, Austin, TX 78714. Phone: (512) 926-4900; Web site: herbalgram.org.

The Herb Quarterly, 1041 Shary Circle, Concord, CA 94518. Web site: herbquarterly.com.

The Lark Letter, 7811 Montrose Road, Potomac, MD 20854. Web site: drlark.com; E-mail: letters@drlark.com.

Yoga International. Phone: (800) 253-6243; Web site: himalayaninstitute.org.

Yoga Journal, 2054 University Ave., Berkeley, CA 94704. Phone: (800) 600-9642; Web site: yogajournal.com.

ASSOCIATIONS AND WEB SITES

The following organizations provide more detailed information on a variety of health issues and conditions.

American Botanical Council (ABC), P.O. Box 201660, Austin, TX 78720. Phone: (512) 926-4900; Web site: herbalgram.org.

Herb Research Foundation, 1007 Pearl St., #200, Boulder, CO 80302. Phone: (303) 449-2265; Web site: herbs.org.

National Black Woman's Health Project, 1211 Connecticut Ave. NW, #310, Washington, DC 20036. Phone: (202) 835-0117; Web site: nbwhp.org.

National Institute of Mental Health, NIMH Public Inquiries, 6001 Executive Blvd., Rm. 8184, MSC 9663, Bethesda, MD 20892-966. Phone: (301) 443-4513; Web site: nimh.nih.gov; E-mail: nimhinfo@nih.gov.

National Osteoporosis Foundation, 1232 22nd St. NW, Washington, DC 20037. Phone: (202) 223-2226; Web site: nof.org.

Osteoporosis and Women's Health. Web site: osteoporosis-and-womens-health.com.

Osteoporosis Education Project: Rethinking Osteoporosis, 605 Franklin Park Dr., East Syracuse, NY 13057. Phone: (315) 437-9384; Web site: betterbones.com; E-mail: info@betterbones.com.

Women's Health Initiative (WHI), 1 Rockledge Center, Suite 300, MS 7966, Bethesda, MD 20892. Phone: (301) 402-2900; Web site: hhlbi.nih.gov/whi. (The National Institutes of Health established WHI in 1991 to study the most common causes of death, disability, and impaired quality of life in postmenopausal women. These studies of 167,000 women will look at the efficacy of hormone replacement therapy, diet, and vitamin supplementation, as well as attempt to identify predictors of disease and understand community approaches to healthful behavior.)

Women's International Pharmacy, 5708 Monona Dr., Madison, WI 54716. Phone: (800) 279-5708; Web site: womensinternational.com; E-mail: info@womensinternational.com.

VIDEOS, AUDIOTAPES, AND OTHER PRODUCTS

Videos

AM and PM Yoga for Beginners with Rodney Yee and Patricia Walden (two-volume set).

Flowing Yoga Postures for Beginners with Lilias Folan.

Prenatal Yoga with Colette Crawford.

Prenatal Yoga with Shiva Rea.

Yoga for Round Bodies (volumes 1 and 2) with Linda DeMarco and Genia Pauli Haddon.

Yoga Journal's Practice Series:

> *Yoga Practice: Introduction* with Patricia Walden
> *Yoga Practice for Beginners* with Patricia Walden
> *Yoga Practice for Flexibility* with Patricia Walden
> *Yoga Practice for Strength* with Rodney Yee
> *Yoga Practice for Relaxation* with Patricia Walden and Rodney Yee
> *Yoga Practice for Energy* with Rodney Yee
> *Yoga Practice for Meditation* with Rodney Yee

Audiotapes

Discover Yoga with Lilias Folan.
Discover Serenity with Lilias Folan.

Products

The following mail-order companies offer a variety of items that may help you with your yoga practice, including yoga mats, blankets, blocks, bolsters, straps, inversion aids, and even clothing. Contact companies directly to find out what they carry.

Body Lift. Phone: (888) 243-3279; Web site: ageeasy.com.

Hugger Mugger Yoga Products. Phone: (800) 473-4888;
Web site: huggermugger.com.

Lilias products. naturaljourneys.com.

Living Arts catalog. Phone: (800) 254-8464; Web site: gaiam.com.

Tools for Yoga. Phone: (888) 678-9642; Web site: yogapropshop.com.

Yoga Accessories. Phone: (800) 990-9642; Web site: yogaaccessories.com.

Yoga Mats. Phone: (800) 720-9642; Web site: yogamats.com.

YogaPro. Phone: (800) 488-6414; Web site: yogapro.com.

Yoga Props. Phone: (888) 856-9642; Web site: yogaprops.net.

Yoga Shop 4U. Phone: (401) 353-3513; Web site: yogashop4u.com.

Yoga Wear. Phone: (800) 217-0006; Web site: www.mariewright.net.

Acknowledgments

I HAVE LOTS OF PEOPLE TO THANK FOR HELPING ME MAKE THIS book a reality. Of course, the first person on my list is Patricia Walden. I feel so blessed having her as my teacher, my writing partner, and above all, my friend. Besides painstakingly creating the sequences, Patricia shared her wisdom and her vast experience in yoga and women's health, and helped me balance the stress of researching and writing with a healthy dose of humor. I have a deep sense of gratitude for the work of B. K. S. Iyengar, a modern-day yogi and therapeutic genius, and his daughter, Geeta, who is clearly a pioneer in the field of women's health and yoga. Patricia's inspiration and teachings come from her close association with the Iyengars; without their groundbreaking work, this book (like so many others) would simply not be possible.

Annie Carpenter—what a gem! She deserves a very special thank-you for selflessly taking so much time out of her crazy teaching schedule to fly up to San Francisco and spend time talking about bones. In fact, we shared hours and hours of "bone-speak." She provided the sequences for hyper-kyphosis and osteoporotic breaks and spoke so affectionately of the women she's worked with; her enthusiasm was truly infectious. By the time she left for Los Angeles, I had reams of notes and a new friendship.

Thanks also to Gail Greendale, M.D., of UCLA who spent more time than I'm sure she could afford talking about yoga and hyperkyphosis; Sylvia Unger, the oldest participant in Gail and Annie's kyphosis study, who continues to do yoga "in her mind" and who so willingly gave me an insider's perspective; and Susan E. Brown, Ph.D., who patiently put osteoporosis into a historical perspective for me and graciously wrote the foreword.

I am forever indebted to the publishing cast who believed in this project from the very beginning: my agent, Joe Spieler, along with Peter Turner and Jonathan Green at Shambhala Publications, took care of all the details; copy editors extraordinaire Jim Keough and Karen Steib made me sound much better than I should; designers Steve Dyer and Greta Sibley created a beautiful product; and publicist Peter Bermudes made sure the whole world saw it. Absolutely everyone should have an editor like Emily Bower—she pushed me when I got stuck and held my hand (from Boston to California) when I needed encouragement, all the while making sure we met our deadlines.

I'm so lucky to get to work with yoga photographer David Martinez again. I thank him from the bottom of my heart for his patience and his unflappability (if that's even a word!) and his choice of assistants, Aneata Ferguson and Charlie Nucci. I am so grateful to Eleanor Williams and Catherine de los Santos. Both of these lovely yoginis put their own lives and teaching schedules on hold to model the beautiful poses you see in these pages. Brenda Beebe, owner of Yoga Mats in San Francisco, is also a good friend who generously provided all the props featured in the sequences.

I'm thankful to all the teachers who work with me at the San Francisco Bay Club and Bay Club Marin for listening to me carry on about bones month after month—especially Lee Monozon, Leigh Threlkel, Amy Stone, and my lovely assistant, Erin Peary, who kept things running when I was hiding out at my computer. Thanks to Nestor Fernandez and Jim Gerber, my "bosses," who gave me time off to write, and to my writing buddies, Stephen Cope, Kathryn Arnold, and Anne Cushman, who believed in me no matter what. Above all, I want to honor my teachers—Patricia Sullivan, Sarah Powers, Sharon Gannon, Bri. Maya Tiwari, Marion Woodman, Ty Powers, Sharon Salzberg, Patty Craves, and Janice Gates. They have contributed more than they know to my own understanding of this deep and abiding practice, and they have singly and collectively held me in their hearts and contributed greatly to my own healing.

Finally, I would never have completed this book without the love and support I get at home, especially from my husband and on-site editor, Jim Keough. Although our daughters, Sarah and Megan, are no longer living nearby, their cheerleading from across the miles kept me going, and their invitations to visit provided the right amount of distraction. *Yoga for Healthy Bones* is clearly a community project. If I have neglected to list someone by name, please know I'll find you soon enough in my heart and shout a heartfelt thank-you for all the world to hear.

Index